GENETIC ORIGINS OF TUMOR CELLS

DEVELOPMENTS IN ONCOLOGY

VOLUME 1

2. J. Aisner and P. Chang, eds. Cancer Treatment Research.
ISBN 90-247-2358-2

GENETIC ORIGINS
OF TUMOR CELLS

edited by

F.J. CLETON M.D.
The Netherlands Cancer Institute, Amsterdam

and

J.W.I.M. SIMONS Ph.D.
Laboratory for Radiation Genetics and Chemical Mutagenesis, Leiden

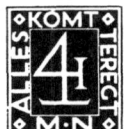

1980

MARTINUS NIJHOFF PUBLISHERS
THE HAGUE / BOSTON / LONDON

Distributors:

for the United States and Canada

Kluwer Boston, Inc.
160 Old Derby Street
Hingham, MA 02043
USA

for all other countries

Kluwer Academic Publishers Group
Distribution Center
P.O. Box 322
3300 AH Dordrecht
The Netherlands

Library of Congress Cataloging in Publication Data   CIP

Main entry under title:

Genetic origins of tumor cells.

    (Developments in oncology; v.1)
    1. Cancer — Genetic aspects. 2. Cancer cells. 3. Carcinogenesis. I. Cleton,
F.J. II. Simons, J.W.I.M. III. Series.
RC268.4.G45   616.9'92'071   79-22440

ISBN-13:978-94-009-8825-5   e-ISBN-13:978-94-009-8823-1
DOI: 10.1007/978-94-009-8823-1

CONTENTS

PREFACE

In 1978 the *Dutch Genetic Society* organized a symposium on the genetic aspects of the origin of tumor cells. The objective of this symposium was to reach an overview of the state of knowledge in a number of quite different fields related to each other through the genetics of the initiation of tumor cells.

This monograph contains the brought-up-to-date contributions of this symposium. Herein discussed is the extent that characteristics of tumor cells can be considered as a phenotype. The possible role of somatic mutation and repair of genetic damage is studied and the analysis of genes with oncogenic potential is pursued. Also the influence of host factors in the response to oncogenic action is dealt with.

This volume describes in a clear and concise manner the current status in these research areas and, it is hoped, will stimulate the exchange of information and ideas between them.

Dr. F.J. CLETON,
The Netherlands Cancer Institute, Amsterdam

Dr. J.W.I.M. SIMONS,
Department of Radiation Genetics and Chemical Mutagenesis,
University of Leiden

CONTRIBUTORS

P. Bentvelzen Ph.D.
Radiobiological Institute TNO, Lange Kleiweg 151, Rijswijk (ZH), The Netherlands.

F.J. Cleton M.D.
Antoni van Leeuwenhoek-Huis, The Netherlands Cancer Institute, Plesmanlaan 121, Amsterdam, The Netherlands.

P. Démant M.D.
Antoni van Leeuwenhoek-Huis, The Netherlands Cancer Institute, Plesmanlaan 121, Amsterdam, The Netherlands.

A.J. van der Eb Ph.D., H. Jochemsen, J.H. Lupker, J. Maat, H. van Ormondt, P.I. Schrier.
Laboratory for Physiological Chemistry, Sylvius Laboratories Leiden University, Wassenaarseweg 72, Leiden. The Netherlands.

B.W. Glickman Ph.D.
Department of Molecular Genetics, Leiden University, Wassenaarseweg 64, Leiden, The Netherlands.

G.R. Mohn Ph.D.
Department of Radiation Genetics and Chemical Mutagenesis, Leiden University, Wassenaarseweg 72, Leiden, The Netherlands.

Th.G. van Rijssel M.D.
Department of Pathology Anatomy, Leiden University, Wassenaarseweg 62, Leiden, The Netherlands.

R.A. Schilperoort Ph.D., P.M. Klapwijk, G. Ooms, G.J. Wullems
Department of Biochemistry, Leiden University, P.O. Box 9505, Leiden, The Netherlands.

J.W.I.M. Simons Ph.D.
Department of Radiation Genetics and Chemical Mutagenesis, Leiden University, Wassenaarseweg 72, Leiden, The Netherlands.

L.A. Smets Ph.D.
Antoni van Leeuwenhoek-Huis, The Netherlands Cancer Institute, Plesmanlaan 121, Amsterdam, The Netherlands.

INTRODUCTION ON THE GENESIS OF TUMOUR CELLS

TH.G. VAN RIJSSEL

The phenomenon of tumour growth — or neoplasia — is a general risk in the life cycle of multicellular organisms, and has been studied on several widely different levels, reaching from world-wide population studies to research on molecular changes in cancer cells. At all these levels fundamental observations have been made and some will be mentioned here as introduction.

1. POPULATION LEVEL

The incidence of cancer in human populations varies markedly, in close relation to the mean expectation of life, as many of the common types of cancer occur mainly in the oldest age groups. In the Netherlands 25% of the annual mortality is due to cancer and one from every three inhabitants will be hit by a form of this disease.

Epidemiologic studies have demonstrated that the incidence of cancer varies greatly in different geographic areas and also in different socioeconomic layers. It is possible to identify *risk-factors* for certain tumour types in this way.

2. PATIENT LEVEL

Cancer is not one clinical disease entity. The syndromes caused by tumours are very polymorphous and depend in the first place on the tumour site, which can be any part of the body.

Local changes may be deformation, compression, obstruction and destruction, leading to impairment of organ functions. General signs may be cachexia, fever, and other systemic effects, including immunological reactions. Identification of the type and the extension of the tumour, and of the absence or presence of metastasis are indispensable for decision on optimal treatment.

F.J. Cleton and J.W.I.M. Simons (eds.), Genetic Origins of Tumor Cells. IX—XVI.
Copyright © 1980 by Martinus Nijhoff Publishers bv, The Hague/Boston/London.
All rights reserved.

3. TUMOUR LEVEL

There are hundreds of tumour types, with different behaviour, structure and etiology, occurring in each tissue of the body, causing different clinical syndromes with diverging course, and each requiring a treatment adapted to the special features of the case. Tumour types with the potential of spreading through the body are called *malignant*. It is now a good hundred years ago that the phenomenon of spreading or *metastasis* was recognized as autotransplantation of cells disseminated from the primary tumour. Malignant tumour cells invade surrounding tissues, lymphatic vessels and small veins; they are transported with lymph or blood to lymph nodes or other organs. These embolic tumour cells may penetrate into the surrounding tissue, settle there, multiply and form a colony, growing out into secondary or metastatic tumour.

Cancer is the comprehensive name for all malignant tumours; however the grade of malignancy in various types of cancer varies greatly. In types with a high grade of malignancy numerous metastases develop early, i.e. when the primary tumour is still small. Other tumour types have a low potential for invasive growth and dissemination, metastases only develop late and in a small number; their grade of malignancy is low. Tumour types which do not metastasize at all are not cancerous and are called *benign*. Notwithstanding the great variation in behaviour and morphology of tumour types, all neoplasms have one characteristic in common: *continuous growth*, which is harmful for the organism. Nearly all human tissues contain cells able to multiply, as can be demonstrated by explanting tissue fragments in vitro under suitable conditions. These cells are mainly the stem cells, reserve cells or germinative cells which give the tissues their regenerative capacity. These cells do not divide when no replacement of lost cells or regenerative activity is required, and, when the tissue has been damaged, their multiplication is strictly controlled. In regenerative proliferation a cell division usually is followed by differentiation of one of the daughter cells, while the other one stays a germinative cell; when the number of differentiated cells has been filled up, mitotic activity ends. Tumour cells differ from normal cells in the tissues by continuous proliferation which is evidently not controlled by the normal regulation mechanism; the growth of tumours is *autonomous*.

4. CELLULAR LEVEL

One of the fundamental problems in oncology is why tumour cells are insensitive to the normal regulation of cell proliferation and growth. Why do the signals which suppress mitotic activity in the tissues have no inhibitory effect on tumour cells? Where is the interruption of the information chain via the receptors on the cell surface to the mitosis-preparing apparatus in the tumour cell?

The mitotic cycle of tumour cells does not usually take less time than in normal cells. Tumour growth is not mainly based on acceleration of the mitotic cell-cycle, but on a lack of maturation of the tumour cells. After mitosis of a tumour cell *both* daughter cells will prepare for a new mitosis, etc., etc., and their differentiation is less than in normal tissue. The less the grade of differentiation, the higher the grade of malignancy.

Cancer cells only stop their reproduction and growth when no sufficient supply for synthesis is available, as is often the case in central areas of larger tumours because the tissue architecture is less efficient in tumours than in normal organs. Such a tumour shows a necrotic centre and an actively growing periphery.

Much research has been performed to find abnormalities of structure or metabolism of tumour cells which could make their abnormal behaviour understandable.

Several abnormalities of tumour cells have been described. They may show irregularities of DNA content and chromatin arrangement, aneuploidy and chromosomal abnormalities and changes of the plasma membrane which may contain, among others, unusual glycopeptids.

Normal cells show contact inhibition in vitro, i.e. when their surface comes in contact with another cell they stop moving in that direction and do not prepare for cell division. Cancer cells have lost this contact inhibition and move in vitro actively across other cells, continuing their growth and piling up several layers of cells, producing a multilayer culture instead of a monolayer.

Cancer cells are also less cohesive and show in vitro less adhesion than normal cells of similar type. These properties probably result from abnormalities of their cell surface and are considered to contribute to their capacity for infiltrating growth and metastatic spread.

The appearance of neoantigens on the cell surface is another manifestation of changes in the plasma membrane. Some of these neoantigens are similar to embryonal antigens which are normally produced in certain cells of the foetus. This production stops at the end of the prenatal period and the genetic information for that production subsequently remains masked. The reappearance of these antigens in the cell surface of tumour cells is considered to be the result of the demasking of these genes. The same holds for the production of peptid hormone fragments by tumours of cell types normally never producing such hormones. Neoantigens in tumour cells which are really new have to be considered as resulting from changes of genes, or from addition of new genetic information (as in viral tumours). It is evident that the regulation of gen activity in tumour cells is impaired in several ways.

5. ETIOLOGY

In the first years of the 20th century the main objective of oncological research was to find the cause of cancer. In the search for carcinogenic (= cancerogenic) agents it became clear that many quite heterogenous factors could be responsible for the development of tumours.

— U-V *radiation* proved to be the main causal factor in carcinogenesis in human skin, and ionizing irradiation was recognized as carcinogenic for the skin and deeper tissues.
— After Rous' discovery in 1911 that cell-free filtrate of chicken sarcoma was cancerogenic, several *oncogenic viruses* have been identified, of both DNA and RNA type. In the 1960s the first indications were found for viral factors in some human tumours.
— More than 100 years after Pott's discovery that soot and tar were responsible for the scrotal skin cancer of chimney sweeps, the first skin tumours were induced experimentally with tar. After the identification and isolation of potent *cancerogenic chemicals* (polycyclic hydrocarbons) the study of the early phases of tumour development began. Several chemicals of very different structure were found to be carcinogenic (e.g. aromatic amines, nitrosamines, amino-azodyes, alkylating agents, aflatoxin).
— In certain situations hyperstimulation by proliferation inducing *hormones* leads to tumour growth in the target tissue.
— A surprising observation was that inert substances (polymers or metals), when implanted in rats as thin films, induced sarcomas in the fibrous tissue layer which had been formed as encapsulation of the implant. When the substance was administered in powder form or as a film with perforations, no tumours arose. Evidently the physical presence and the continuous cleavage of the tissues over a large area formed a carcinogenic stimulus (*solid state* carcinogenesis).

– Diet, genetic constitution (histocompatibility genes) and some immune functions proved to be *modifying factors* in the experiments.

The general conclusion from the investigations on the etiology of cancer is that the induction of tumour growth is accomplished by a constellation of influences, some carcinogenic, others cocarcinogenic, enhancing, inhibiting, modifying, exogenous as well as endogenous.

6. CARCINOGENESIS

The discovery of carcinogenic chemicals made it possible to study their effect in the tissues and to follow the development of tumour growth.

Some important results were obtained with experiments on carcinogenesis in the skin, two of which results are summarized here:

1. The first change in the skin after a low dose of a carcinogen was epidermal hyperplasia which disappeared after some time. When more doses were given the hyperplasia was more marked with tumourlike areas; these areas were irreversibly changed, but did not grow further.
2. When still more carcinogen was applied, tumour growth developed and persisted, even without any further application of the carcinogen.

This experiment shows that carcinogenesis is a stepwise process:

phase 1 – only reversible hyperplasia was observed;
phase 2 – an irreversible non progressive hyperplastic tumourlike state (conditional tumour) had been produced;
phase 3 – real autonomous tumour growth had developed and continued.

Berenblum demonstrated that even a dose of carcinogen which was too small to cause tumour growth has a lasting effect on the skin. When, after application of such a subeffective dose, he treated the same area of the skin repeatedly with irritating substances (which did not induce tumour growth in non-pretreated skin), severe epidermal damage and regeneration were provoked and after some months tumours developed. He concluded that the low dose carcinogen had caused an irreversible change (= initiation) in some cells which stayed "dormant" until they were awakened and forced into proliferation by the skin damage "promoting" substance. In this proliferation some of the initiated cells completed their development into full cancer cells.

These experiments suggest that the transformation of normal cells into cancer cells is not a sudden event like being struck by lightning, but a stepwise process of successive changes, each leading to a following discrete phase until the transformation is complete and the cells have all the characteristics of cancer cells.

Several observations on human tumours are also compatible with the concept that carcinogenesis is a multiphase process.

— Many patients with chronic affections have an increased risk of developing cancer. Examples are polyposis of colon, solar keratosis of the skin, multiple exostoses of the skeleton, etc. In these affections, which are called *precancerous*, proliferative alterations are present which do not show the characteristics of tumour growth, but have a predisposition to acquire these.
— Other patients have local epithelial lesions with the microscopical characteristics of carcinoma but without any invasive growth or metastasis. These lesions, called *carcinoma in situ*, also have a high risk of becoming fully carcinomatous after some years.
— It is not unusual that in human tumours of low malignancy a new cell clone develops after some time which grows faster, with shorter mitotic cycle and less differentiation. Such a clone which may overgrow the other cells has a higher tendency to metastasis. This increase of malignancy is called *progression*. In this way e.g. a slowly growing cartilaginous tumour may give rise to an aggressive fibrosarcoma of high malignancy.

These examples illustrate that in human pathology also indications may be found that cancer develops stepwise via discrete stages.

It is now generally accepted that carcinogenesis begins with some change in the information-carrying macromolecules of the cell and there is strong evidence that the initiating lesion is usually located in DNA molecules.

When the DNA damage is not repaired, an irreversible alteration remains which will be present in the daughter cells; the changes in cell behaviour resulting from this lesion of the genome can be considered as *somatic mutations*. Indeed, mutagenesis studies have shown that many, and perhaps all, carcinogenic substances are mutagenic. The introduction of new nuclear acids in persistent infection with oncovirus is analogous with mutations.

Complete carcinogens are able to induce this initiation as well as the further changes leading to the growth of cancer. Some substances are called incomplete carcinogens: a few can only induce the initiating lesion, but no further steps (initiators); other substances are not able to induce initiation but can provoke further steps and this action is called cocarcinogenic (e.g. promotors). When a carcinogenic agent has induced the first imprint in the genetic material of one or more cells, an unknown number of further changes have to take place before cells will grow autonomously. When the initiated cells do not proliferate, no consequences of the hit will become manifest. Influences which stimulate cell proliferation in tissues with initiated cells often have a cocarcinogenic action; indeed all promoting substances provoke much reactive cell proliferation. Also stimulation by hormonal action, regeneration after (viral) infections or repeated mechanical trauma may result in increased cell production with a cocarcinogenic effect. In this proliferation, dividing initiated cells show a loss of differentiation potential and after several divisions more defects may result from the original genetic damage. Some of the irreversible effects may be epigenetic, i.e. based on a changed expression of the genetic information.

When tissues containing such precursor cancer cells are hit again by a carcinogenic or cocarcinogenic agent, new steps of the carcinogenetic process can be made and in this way successively all the characteristics of tumour growth are obtained and progression to highly malignant cancer takes place.

It has been demonstrated in several model systems that when carcinogenic influences of different kinds act upon the same tissue their effect is cumulative (syncarcinogenesis). The latent period between the first contact with carcinogenic agents and the appearance of tumour growth varies widely. In experiments with oncogenic viruses in mice this period may be some weeks; observations in man suggest that the development of tumour growth may take more than half a century.

It is reasonable to suppose that all human beings are exposed during their whole lifetime to many different carcinogenic agents. Burnet has suggested that mutated cells which are precursors of cancer cells are often eliminated by immunological activity because of the abnormal antigenic structure of their surface. It is not certain whether this mechanism exists, or, if it does, how many incipient tumours are thereby conquered. But in more than 30% of human beings reaching old age this hypothetical immune surveillance apparently fails.

Summarizing we can conclude that:
Tumour growth is continuous proliferation of cells which have lost

their sensitivity for the normal growth-regulating signals and therefore grow autonomously.

Cancer is malignant tumour cell proliferation, characterized by the potential for metastasis.

Cancer is caused by varying constellations of several heterogenous factors which can be classified as carcinogenic, cocarcinogenic and modifying factors.

Carcinogenesis is a complex multistage process. Its first stage is initiation, probably resulting in an irreversible imprint in DNA, which genetic lesion can be considered as somatic mutation. Further development depends on genetic and epigenetic mechanisms, e.g. promotion by cell proliferation-stimulating factors. New hits will cause progression to new stage until finally a cell clone develops with all the characteristics of cancer cells. This autonomously proliferating clone will, after a growth period varying from weeks to years, become a clinically detectable tumour.

1. STABLE PHENOTYPIC EXPRESSIONS OF TRANSFORMED AND TUMOR CELLS

L.A. SMETS

ABSTRACT

In this paper, the genetic aspects of the phenotypic alterations observed in cells after malignant transformation are discussed. A number of discrete and stable phenotypic changes are described which accumulate progressively by a mutation-selection process. This multistep process of cell transformation and tumor induction appears to be modulated by the genetic background of the target cell.

1. INTRODUCTION

There is ample evidence that the cellular genome is involved in the acquisition of the various properties which convert a normal cell into a malignant one. This evidence includes the well-known correspondence between mutagenic and carcinogenic properties of various chemicals or the incorporation of viral genomes (or their subsequent activation) as a fundamental step in the pathogenesis of virus-induced tumors. Moreover, the presence of specific chromosomal aberrations in some malignant diseases or in conditions at risk for tumor development has been documented in some cases, most notably human leukemia.

A fundamental and most frequently posed question is whether neoplastic transformation is genetic in nature or epigenetic. In other words, whether the relevant changes disturb the one-dimensional arrangement in DNA sequence or whether they relate to changes in the coordinated expression, the "editing", of otherwise unchanged information.

Cancer appears as a social disorder of cells and is invariably associated with disturbance of normal differentiation. Moreover, its causation is often multifactoral and tumor development proceeds through many qualitatively different steps. It is evident that such complex processes are difficult to explain by the concepts derived from microbial and Mendelian genetics.

F.J. Cleton and J.W.I.M. Simons (eds.), Genetic Origins of Tumor Cells. 1–10.
Copyright © 1980 by Martinus Nijhoff Publishers bv, The Hague/Boston/London.
All rights reserved.

To close the gap between the phenomenology of disturbed growth control on the one hand and the responsible molecular changes at the genetic level on the other hand, one should be able to define at least a number of stable and discrete phenotypic changes in tumor cells which presumably are directly derived from hereditary changes. In this paper, an attempt is made to select and describe the most prominent phenotypic changes associated with transformed and tumor cells and to outline their various interrelationships.

2. PHENOTYPIC CHANGES IN TRANSFORMED AND TUMOR CELLS

Numerous changes have been described in cells transformed in tissue culture by chemical, physical or viral determinants (Nicolson, 1974; Pontén, 1976). Most of these changes are also observed in tumor cells explanted in tissue culture. In addition, tumor cells in vivo display a number of properties not present in (or not expressed by) tissue culture cells. The following summary — although not arbitrary — will be of necessity incomplete.

2.1. Changes in social behaviour

The most prominent change observed in tissue culture concerns the social behaviour of transformed and tumor cells. Normal cells are subjected to a type of growth control known as *contact inhibition*. Contact between normal cells causes the cessation of their motile behaviour followed by a reversal of the direction of movement (Abercrombie and Heaysman, 1954). In crowded cultures, the increased degree of intercellular contact imposes a growth restraint on the cells. The ultimate effect of contact inhibition is the formation of an ordered monolayer of quiescent, nondividing cells. Transformed cells, on the other hand, do not respond or respond less effectively to this type of growth control and develop into multilayered cultures of irregularly ordered cells growing on top of each other. In these cultures growth will be restrained only by inadequate nutrient supply and the accumulation of waste products.

Transformed cells also differ in the *decreased requirement* for certain factors in the serum complement of the culture medium. They can grow at serum concentrations too low to support the growth of normal cells and in some cases even in completely synthetic media.

Another alteration observed in many transformed and most tumor-derived cells is their ability to grow while suspended in semi-solid media containing agarose or methyl cellulose (Stoker et al., 1968). Normal cells will not proliferate under these conditions, since they require attachment or anchorage to a substrate for growth. Some transformed and most tumor cells, however, are able to form spherical colonies in suspension. The acquisition of this property after transformation is known as *anchorage independence*.

Probably the most meaningful change in the social behaviour of transformed cells is the capacity of *infinite growth*. According to the concept of Hayflick (1965), normal cells are programmed for a varying but limited number of divisions. In consequence, normal cells have a finite life-span and cultures of such cells will die out sooner or later depending on the tissue of origin and the age of the donor. In contrast, transformed and explanted tumor cells are capable of infinite growth. An intermediate situation is encountered with so-called established cell lines of untransformed cells. In these cells — mainly derived from rodent animals — a normal phenotype is preserved in cells with infinite life-span. However, these established cell lines are not normal since they show chromosomal aneuploidy and can rapidly transform spontaneously. Mouse 3T3 cells and hamster BHK cells are examples of such established, untransformed cells. In contrast, established cell lines can not be made from normal cells of avian or human origin. Cultures of such cells remain diploid and die out after a given number of cell divisions. Spontaneous transformation is never observed in these cells, which have to be treated with carcinogenic agents to acquire an infinite growth potential. These observations point to the rôle of the genetic background in the transformation behaviour of cells of different origin, as will be discussed later.

2.2. Changes in membrane properties

Although the primary changes responsible for (tumorigenic) transformation are located in the cell genome, many of these changes must express themselves as alterations at the cell surface. Numerous studies have indicated that the cell membrane is the organelle primarily involved in the social interactions of cells. In consequence, a social disorder at the cellular level such as cancer will be accompanied by changes at or near the cell membrane.

Several reviews summarize the alterations in membrane properties observed in transformed and tumor-derived cells (Nicolson, 1976; Smith and Walburg, 1977). Figure 1 summarizes in a schematic way a number of these alterations, some of which refer to the changes in

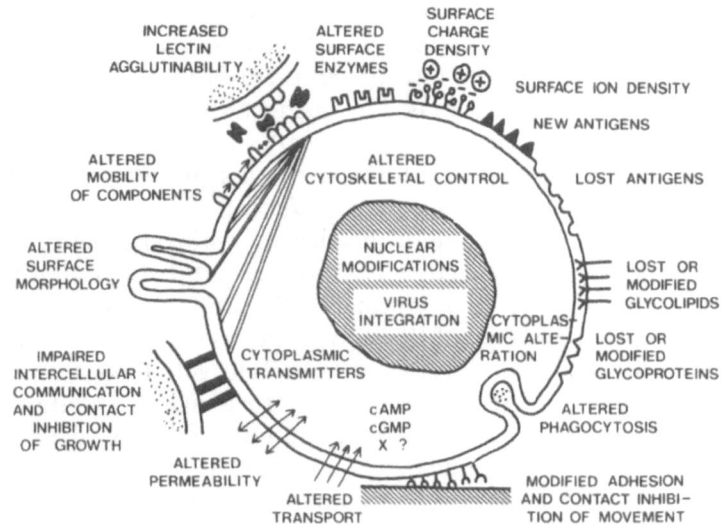

Figure 1. Diagramatic representation of the various changes observed at or near the surface of tumor cells (modified by J. Collard after Robbins and Nicolson).

the social behaviour already described in the previous paragraphs.

A particular change in membrane properties of transformed and tumor cells is the *increased agglutinability* with plant lectins such as Concanavalin A (Nicolson, 1974). This property monitors a change in surface architecture of the transformed cell surface. As the factors involved are manifold and complex, the phenomenon remains as yet largely unexplained.

Among the changes in the amount or composition of membrane components, those concerning membrane glycoproteins deserve further attention. Membrane glycoproteins are embedded with their globulin protein part in the membrane lipid bilayer. The hydrophylic part, carrying the carbohydrate units, extends into the cell exterior. These carbohydrate units are considered to act as antennae which receive signals from the environment as well as from neighbouring cells. It has been postulated that the membrane glycoproteins trans-duce these signals through the membrane into the cell interior (Nicolson, 1976). A *structural change in membrane glycoprotein* has been reported as a general accompaniment of tumorigenic transforma-tion (Van Beek et al., 1975, 1978). This change, illustrated in Figure 2, manifests itself by an increased molecular weight of membrane glycopeptides due to the presence of extra sialic acids or other

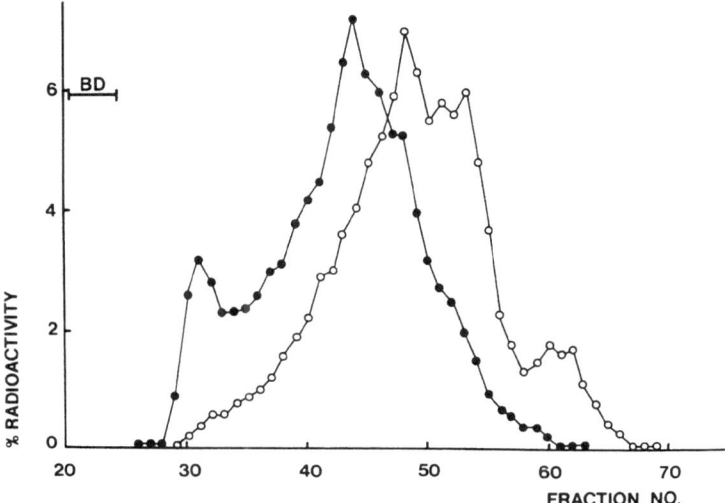

Figure 2. Gelfiltration elution profile of fucose-labeled membrane glycopeptides from mouse mammary tumor (black circles) compared with glycopeptides from normal mammary gland (open circles). The malignant glycopeptides elute in front of control material indicating increased molecular weight distribution.

negatively charged terminal groups of the carbohydrate units. Its biological function remains obscure but no correlation with the changes in social behaviour of cells in tissue culture has been found. On the other hand, the correlation of this biochemical change with malignancy is high, if not absolute (Smets et al. 1976, 1977).

2.3. Changes in tumor cells in situ

In addition to the various alterations observed in tissue culture, tumor cells display many deviations from normal when observed in vivo. Tumor cells escape from various types of growth, positional and immunological control. In addition, tumors may develop the capacity to metastasize, that is, to nestle and grow in foreign and distant organs. During treatment, tumor cells may develop resistance to the drugs used.

Most of these properties are less well circumscribed than those observed with transformed cells in tissue culture. Some properties of tumor cells are probably also expressed after explantation in tissue culture; for instance, the capacity of uncontrolled and infinite growth. Other properties, however, may not have corresponding phenomena in

vitro. This situation certainly pertains for the escape from immunological control or the capacity for metastasis.

For the present discussion it is sufficient to state that tumor cells
in situ have acquired a number of changes in addition to those
observed in transformed cells in tissue culture.

3. CORRELATION BETWEEN VARIOUS CHANGES

It is evident that the manifold changes accompanying cell transformation can not be dealt with as heriditary changes unless some criteria
have been met. Therefore, it is suggested here to "filter" the vast
amount of data using the following criteria:

1. Any change in transformed or tumor-derived cells should be general
   in nature and not a specific property of certain cell types only, i.e.
   fibroblasts or lymphoid cells.
2. The changes should be primary and not secondary changes resulting
   from differences in growth rate or cell density.
3. Pleiotypic changes should be combined into a single change, probably related to a common hereditary alteration.

The analysis of pleiotypic expressions is most adequately executed
by investigating clonal cell lines isolated from transformed cell
cultures. Properties which do not segregate in the variant cell lines can
then be considered as pleiotypic expressions (compare Smets et al.,
1976).

The outcome of this filtering process is summarized in Table I,
which shows a number of alterations observed in transformed cells

Table 1. Stable phenotypic changes in transformed cells.

Change	Associated changes	Tumori-genicity[a]
1. Infinite life-span	growth related changes	5.10^7
2. Morphological transformation	increased agglutination decreased contact inhibition decreased serum requirement	10^6
3. Anchorage independence	fibrinolytic activity	10^4
4. Membrane glycopr. changes	none known	$<10^3$

[a] Average nr. of cells required to produce tumors in rodents.

which fulfill the condition for stable and discrete hereditary changes. The progressive accumulation of these properties renders a cell more tumorigenic.

These properties are also correlated in time. Thus, normal cells may acquire the capacity of infinite life-span without being morphologically transformed. Morphological transformation can be induced in normal or untransformed cells which subsequently may progress to a state of anchorage independence. Eventually, tumor-specific changes in membrane glycopeptides appear in the tumors induced by injection of transformed cells.

Finally, the occurrence of the alterations listed in Table 1 may also be correlated with the amount of viral DNA incorporated by cells infected with fragments of oncogenic genomes. As outlined by Van der Eb (1980), small fragments of Adenovirus DNA induce infinite life-span in normal rat kidney cells. Fragments of larger size, however, are capable of the additional induction of morphological transformation. Transformation with intact virions, e.g. with Polyoma virus, can result in cells showing anchorage-independence as well as membrane glycoprotein changes.

4. CELL TRANSFORMATION AND TUMOR FORMATION

As outlined in the previous paragraphs, tumor cells in vivo have acquired a number of phenotypic changes in addition to those observed in transformed cells. Therefore, cells transformation represents only a few steps of the multistep process of tumor formation. This conclusion is not invalidated by the fact that injection of transformed cells into suitable hosts gives rise to tumors, suggesting that cell transformation alone produces a fully malignant phenotype. It has been demonstrated in various cases that a tumor induced by transformed cells is of monoclonal origin, that is, originates from a single cell contained in the inoculum. Studies with hybrid cells have also indicated that the transformed phenotype is a necessary but not a sufficient condition for the malignant condition (Stanbridge and Wilkinson, 1978), proving that the ability to form tumors is under different genetic control. In line with these findings are the differences in the kinetics of cell transformation as compared with those of tumor induction. Cell transformation often appears as a one-step process, resembling somatic mutation induction. Tumor induction, however, is a multistep process in which many stimulating and permitting factors are involved (Emmelot and Scherer, 1977).

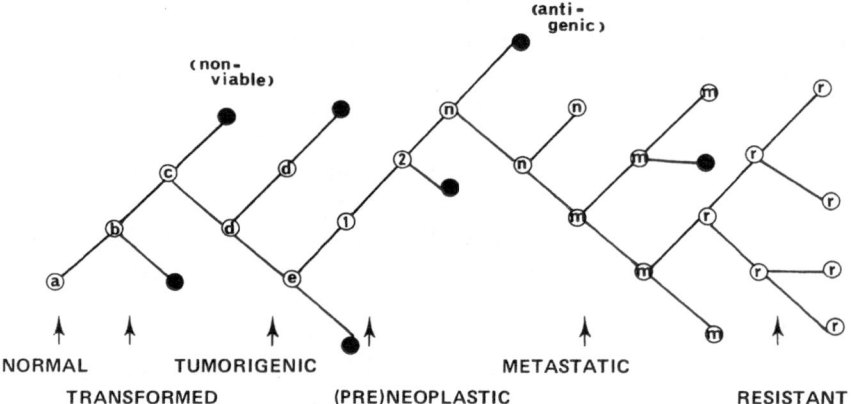

Figure 3. Schematic representation of the clonal origin and the progressive, multi-step development of transformed and tumor cells. The conditions in tissue culture can select for variants with increasing degree of transformation (a-e). Within the host, variant cells are selected with increasing degree of malignancy (1-n), including metastatic (m) and drug-resistant (r) variants. Black circles represent variants with negative selective advantage, e.g. slowly growing or antigenic cells (after Nowell, 1976).

Unlike transformation-dependent changes, the in vivo properties of tumor cells are less well defined as stable and discrete phenotypic expressions of corresponding hereditary changes. Nevertheless, several lines of evidence suggest that tumors develop by a progressive process which is based on a selection-mutation mechanism (Nowell, 1976). This concept is illustrated in Figure 3.

It is evident from this scheme that the genetic background of the cells or the animals studied for transformation or tumor induction can markedly interfere with a mutation-selection process. For instance, various laboratory animals may differ in the effectiveness of their DNA repair mechanisms (compare Glickman, 1980) or in the metabolic activation of potentially carcinogenic substances. In addition, the contribution of histocompatibility factors in tumor frequency is well documented (Cleton and Démant, 1980). These and other factors from the genetic background could explain the differences in cell transformation and tumor induction observed not only between various species but also between tissues of the same animal.

5. CONCLUSIONS

The involvement of the cellular genome in (neoplastic) transformation appears at three levels:

1. The interaction of transforming or carcinogenic agents with the genetic material.
2. The progressive accumulation of stable and discrete phenotypic changes by a mutation- selection process.
3. The modulation of these processes by the genetic background of the target cells or animals.

As a consequence, tumor induction is a progressive, multi-factorial and multistep process. Cell transformation, on the other hand, represents only a few steps of this ongoing process (compare Figure 3).

It is well understood that these concepts are derived from generalisations as well as from scattered information. However, the conclusion seems valid that the phenomenology of cell transformation and tumor induction more and more proceeds to the level of being translatable into molecular terms.

REFERENCES

Abercombie, M. and I.E. Heaysman (1954). Observations on the social behavior of cell in tissue culture. II. Monolayering of fibroblasts. Exp. Cell Res. 6: 293–306.
Démant, P. and F.J. Cleton (1980). Histocompatibility genes and neoplasia. This volume, p. 109-125.
Emmelot, P. and E. Scherer (1977). Multi-hit kinetics of tumor formation, with special reference to experimental liver and human lung carcinogenesis and some general conclusions. Cancer Res. 37: 1702-1708.
Glickman, B.W. (1980). DNA-repair and its relationship to the origins of human cancer. This volume, p. 25-51.
Hayflick, L. (1965). The limited in vitro lifetime of human diploid cell strains. Exptl. Cell. Res. 37: 614-636.
Nicolson, G.L. (1974). The interactions of Lectins with animal cell surfaces. Int. Reviews of Cytology 39: 89-190.
Nicolson, G.L. (1976). Trans-membrane control of the receptors on normal and tumor cells. II. Surface changes associated with transformation and malignancy. Biochim. Biophys. Acta 458: 1-72.
Nowell, P.C. (1976). The clonal evolution of tumor cell populations. Acquired genetic lability permits stepwise selection of variant sublines and underlies tumor progression. Science 194: 23-28.
Pontén, J. (1976). The relationship between in vitro transformation and tumor formation in vivo. Biochim. Biophys. Acta 458: 397-432.
Smets, L.A., W.P. Van Beek and R. van Nie (1977). Membrance glycoprotein changes in primary mammary tumors associated with autonomous growth. Cancer Letters 3: 133-138.
Smets, L.A., W.P. Van Beek and H. van Rooy (1976). Surface glycoproteins and concanavalin-A-mediated agglutinability of clonal variants and tumour cells derived from SV40-virus-transformed mouse 3T3 cells. Int. J. Cancer 18: 462-468.

Smith, D.E. and E.F. Walburg, Jr. (1977). The tumor cell periphery: carbohydrate components. In "Mammalian cell membranes," Vol. 3 Jamieson, G.A. and D.M. Robinson, eds., Boston, Butterwords, pp. 115-146.

Stanbridge, E. and J. Wilkinson (1978). Analysis of malignancy in human cells: Malignant and transformed phenotypes are under separate genetic control. Proc. Natl. Acad. Sci. USA 21: 1466-1469.

Stoker, M., C. O'Neill, S. Berryman and V. Waxman (1968). Anchorage and growth regulation in normal and virus-tranformed cells. Int. J. Cancer 3: 683-693.

Van Beek, W.P., L.A. Smets and P. Emmelot (1973). Increased sialic acid density in surface glycoprotein of transformed and malignant cells — a general phenomenon? Cancer Research 33: 2913-2922.

Van Beek, W.P., L.A. Smets, P. Emmelot, K.J. Roozendaal and H. Behrendt (1978). Early recognition of human leukemia by cell surface glycoprotein changes. Leukemia Res. 2: 163-171.

Van der Eb, A., H. Jochemsen, J.H. Lupker, J. Maat, H. van Ormondt and P.I. Schrier (1980). Structure and functions of adenovirus 5 transformation genes. This volume, p. 73-86.

2. ON THE CORRELATION BETWEEN MUTAGENICITY AND CARCINOGENICITY

G.R. MOHN

ABSTRACT

Current estimations on the importance of environmental factors in the etiology of cancer is summarized with special emphasis on the role of chemical agents. The apparent, empirical high degree of correlation between mutagenicity of chemical substances and their carcinogenic activity has led to the proposal of employing short term mutagenicity tests for detecting carcinogens. Arguments in favour and against a causal relationship between the processes of mutation induction and primary cancer initiation have been reviewed; many data favour a mutational change in DNA as initiating event of cancer but they also stress the primordial importance of cytoplasmic factors in the subsequent steps of cancer progression. It is concluded that mutagenicity tests are of value for qualitatively assessing the potential carcinogenicity of environmental chemicals and that further investigations and developments are necessary to reach a more quantitative and therefore predictive capacity.

1. INTRODUCTION

The rapidly increasing number and amount of chemicals which are in current use in man's environment has led to a variety of questions about their safety. Of particular concern is the hazard of cancer being induced, not only because certain chemicals are carcinogenic in animals (mostly rodents) but also because some environmental compounds unexpectedly exerted genetic (mutagenic) effects in experimental organisms. Boveri's old theory of mutational origin of cancer (see Wolf, 1974) which was refined by Bauer in 1928, has increased in acceptance as a result of recent comparative studies of mutagens and carcinogens and as a result of epidemiological studies which indicate a major contribution of environmental factors (occupation, nutrition, chemicals) to the induction of human cancer. The current

F.J. Cleton and J.W.I.M. Simons (eds.), Genetic Origins of Tumor Cells. 11–24.
Copyright © 1980 by Martinus Nijhoff Publishers bv, The Hague/Boston/London.
All rights reserved.

interest in the correlation between the mutagenic and the carcinogenic potential of chemicals is reflected in a multitude of publications
and in recent extensive reviews of various aspects of the problem
(German, 1974; Montesano et al., 1974; Hiatt et al., 1977; Mulvihill
et al., 1977; Miller, 1978); the present review will, therefore, be
restricted to a few points which briefly summarize: (1) the state of
our understanding of the environmental origin of cancer, (2) the
arguments for and against a causal relation between mutagenicity
and carcinogenicity, and (3) current estimation of the value of
mutagenicity tests as screening tools for detecting cancer causing
agents.

2. ENVIRONMENTAL ORIGINS OF CANCER

That exposure of man to chemicals may be a cause of cancer was
suspected in very early ages. In 1775 the British physician Percival
Pott observed and described in "Chirurgical Observations" an enhanced incidence of scrotum and skin cancer in chimney sweepers
and tar products were soon suspected to be the causative agents since
the exposed persons were asked to wash themselves more often. In
the 19th century tumor formation was observed in persons who came
into contact with paraffin oil, tar, petrol and dyes (von Volkmann,
1875; Bell, 1876; Rehn, 1895). And in 1915, Yamagiwa and Ichikawa
reported the experimental induction of tumors in the rabbit a long
time after the animal's skin had been painted with tar. Later on,
many different classes of chemicals were detected as carcinogens in
experimental animals (see, for example, Clayson 1962; Magee and
Barnes, 1967).

The conclusion that environmental factors including chemicals
are a major cause of human cancer was reached only recently, following a variety of epidemiological studies (Higginson, 1969; Janerick
and Lawerance, 1975; Blot et al., 1977). For example, in a population in the Caspian Littoral of Iran the incidence of oesophageal
cancer is strongly correlated to geographical location (Hormozdiary
et al., 1975); genetic differences in this case can hardly be invoked
as a contributing factor and it is probable that different nutritional
habits are responsible for the large differences in cancer frequencies.
Another striking example of influence of environmental factors was
obtained in studies of stomach and colon cancer mortality rates for
Japanese people living in Japan and those living in California (Dunn,
1975). In this case the dramatic drop in incidence of these kinds of

cancers in the second generation following immigration was attributed to dietary differences in the populations. One further study that is pertinent in this regard is the recently concluded investigation of the World Health Organization into the influence of ingestion of aflatoxins on cancer frequency among inhabitants of African countries. Aflatoxins are naturally occurring compounds produced by certain fungi that contaminate foods in the tropics and these compounds are among the most powerful mammalian carcinogens (Wogan, 1976). The epidemiological study demonstrated that aflatoxins are responsible for the high incidence of primary liver cancer among the members of the Zairian population. Similar conclusions were reached following epidemiological studies for cycasin, diethylstilbestrol, vinyl chloride, 2-naphthylamine, asbestos, polycyclic hydrocarbons and some metallocompounds (IARC, 1972-1978). According to estimations of IARC, some nitroso compounds "should be regarded as if they were carcinogenic to humans" (IARC, Vol. 18, 1978; see also Wang et al., 1978).

Of course, the influence of certain genetic backgrounds on cancer susceptibility is well documented now in man and in experimental animals, as demonstrated by the existence of monogenic syndromes which indicate an important role of genetic traits in susceptibility to certain forms of cancer (see Lynch, 1976; Mulvihill et al., 1977); twin studies, that is, the comparison of onset of cancer in monozygotic and in dizygotic twins, however, have indicated that susceptibility to most common cancer forms is not due to inherited genetic differences. It is also evident now that some cancers are due to primary virus infections (in combination with immunological factors) as recently demonstrated in the case of Epstein-Barr virus as cause of Burkitt's lymphoma (de Thé et al., 1978). But regardless of the mechanism(s) involved, it appears that environmental chemicals play a primordial role in the onset of human cancer.

In search of appropriate methods for detecting potential chemical carcinogens present in the human environment, short term mutagenicity tests using lower organisms gain importance because of their rapidity and the possibility of detecting rare mutational events in large populations by specific selective procedures. The usefulness of microbial tests to detect the mutagenic properties of chemicals is usually accepted now, especially since the recognition that practically all chemicals which are mutagenic in mammals or in cultured mammalian cells (Thompson and Baker, 1973) or in animals such as Drosophila (Vogel and Sobels, 1976) are also mutagenic in suitable strains of microorganisms. These data thus pose the question of to what extent mutagenicity tests are indeed good predictors of the results to be expected in tests for carcinogenic activity in animals.

3. CAUSAL RELATIONSHIP BETWEEN MUTATION AND CANCER?

The answer to this question depends on a connection between the two phenomena at the level of mechanism of induction or initiation. If one considers the possibility of mutation in a somatic cell as the initiating event in tumor formation, then there are several striking similarities between the two phenomena (mutation and cancer initiation). Firstly, as for mutations, cancer initiation is a rare event, as demonstrated by the low spontaneous frequency of malignant transformation in primary and in some secondary cell cultures of mammalian organs (see, for example, Reznikoff et al., 1973; Barrett and Ts'O, 1978), but one has also to consider the very high variation in spontaneous and chemically induced frequency of neoplastic transformation in different cell lines which is not reflected in the frequency of tumor formation in the living animal (Parodi and Brambilla, 1978). Cancer initiation is, further, a stochastic process, i.e. governed by the laws of chance as is the mutational event, and hence even if the frequency of cancer incidence is known with precision it will not be possible to predict which individuals in the population will be affected. The second similarity between mutation and cancer initiation is that the alterations are heritable from one cell generation to another, as clearly demonstrated by the clonal growth of tumor cells which exhibit common "marker" chromosomes (Nowell, 1974; de Grouchy and Turleau, 1974) and common enzymic phenotypes in heterozygous patients (Gartler, 1974; Fialkow, 1977). A third similarity is that a single event in a cancer gene is sufficient to provoke malignant transformation as demonstrated in the case of *onc* genes of DNA and RNA tumor viruses (Bentvelzen, 1978; Van der Eb, 1978) indicating that transforming gene(s) may also exist as a silent, normal part of the genome.

A further similarity between mutation and cancer is the existence of "mutator" genes which show an enhanced frequency of spontaneous tumors of certain types, such as Bloom's syndrome and Xeroderma pigmentosum (see Mulvihill et al., 1977). The enhanced frequency of skin tumors in patients suffering from Xeroderma Pigmentosum, for example, is explained by a genetic deficiency in an enzymatic repair pathway which in normal human beings removes most of the DNA lesions induced by ultraviolet sunlight and which would be responsible for cancer induction (Trosko and Chu, 1975). Analogous well studied defects have been demonstrated in bacteria and other organisms which indicate a primordial role of enzymic repair pathways in the induction of mutation (Glickman, 1978).

DNA as the common target molecule for mutation and cancer induction has been repeatedly postulated and thorough investigations on metabolism of carcinogenic and mutagenic substances indicate that electrophilic metabolites are involved in both phenomena (see Miller, 1978). A product of alkylation of DNA, namely O^6-alkylguanine, has been postulated as responsible for tumor initiation (Rajewsky and Goth, 1976) and for mutation induction (Loveless, 1969, Singer, 1976). Another line of evidence supporting DNA as the molecular target for mutation induction and cancer initiation comes from experiments using Syrian hamster embryo cells (Barrett et al., 1978): Ultraviolet irradiation of these cells pretreated with 5-bromodeoxyuridine resulted in enhanced frequencies of neoplastic transformation; the treatment procedure is likely to give only lesions in DNA (single strand breaks) since 5-BUdR readily absorbs light in this portion (near UV) of the spectrum. In fact the procedures also result in the induction of gene mutations as measured by resistance to thioguanine and ouabain. Clear evidence that pyrimidine dimers induced by UV irradiation can give rise to tumors in experimental animals (fish) has also been presented by Hart et al., 1977: the fact that the carcinogenic effects of UV could be reduced by post-irradiation photo-reactivating light strongly indicates that DNA was the molecule involved in precancerous induction.

What concerns the nature of the presumptive DNA alteration which, ultimately, may lead to malignant transformation and tumor formation, is, as yet, only a matter of speculative reasoning. Of the carcinogenic agents that are also mutagens (X-rays, UV irradiation, chemicals) all induce the two main classes of mutations, namely gene mutations and chromosome aberrations. The specific mutation induction spectrum of certain carcinogens indicate that both frame shift mutations and base pair substitutions can be induced by polycyclic hydrocarbons and by alkylating agents, respectively, thus making a gene or point mutation as causative agent probable. Chromosome aberrations, on the other hand, have been repeatedly shown to be associated with certain tumors and certain forms of cancer, but they seem to be a consequence or an accompanying phenomenon of malignancy rather than its cause (see German, 1974). Another line of reasoning also makes gene mutations more likely to be the primordial cause: comparative studies in several organisms indicate that usually

chromosome aberrations require higher doses of chemical treatment
to be induced than gene mutations, and this has been quantitatively
demonstrated in Drosophila melanogaster, where both genetic effects
can be simultaneously measured (Vogel and Sobels, 1976). Since
chemical induction of cancer, e.g. by dialkylnitrosamines, occurs at
treatment conditions where chromosome aberrations are not detected
(in somatic and in germinal cells), point mutations or small gene
deletion or deficiency remain as potential causative agents. More substantial data to decide which genic mutation is responsible is likely to
arise from studies on the mechanisms of malignant transformation in
isolated oncogenes, such as those present in the malignant stage, e.g.
in tumor viruses, or those silent genes present in the genome which
require transformation through a genetic mechanism (mutation) that
by itself is a multistep process involving induction, fixation, and
phenotypic expression.

Substantial arguments against mutations as the only cause of
chemically induced cancer remain. For example, established carcinogens such as asbestos, plastic films, metallic salts and certain hormones
have not been demonstrated to be mutagenic in tests utilizing a large
number of indicator organisms. This result may be due to differences
in metabolic activities of the various organisms since tests for carcinogenicity are usually not performed using the same species and strains
as the mutagenicity tests. The reverse is also true, i.e. potent mutagens
such as certain aminoacridines are not carcinogenic or only barely so.
However, it should be remembered that individual genes can respond
in rather selective ways to different classes of mutagenic chemicals
(Auerbach, 1976), especially if back-mutations are used as genetic
endpoint.

Further inconsistencies between the process of mutation and cancer
initiation have been described by Mishra et al. (1977). In this study
rat embryo cells were shown to undergo malignant transformation
upon treatment with carcinogens and the frequency was very much
enhanced when the cells were first infected with murine leukemia
virus. However, no enhancement of the frequency of either thioguanine
resistant markers or on mutants to ouabain resistance was detected
in these experiments following treatment with the same virus. Another
indication of differences in the mechanism of mutation and cancer
initiation comes from experiments by McKinnel et al. (1969) using
frog carcinoma cells. Nuclei of these cells were transplanted into frog
eggs, and tadpoles of normal appearance were obtained. This result
indicates either that the carcinoma cells still retain a normal genotype or that the cytoplasm of the normal egg has the ability to

suppress the expression of genetically determined malignancy. Further, Mintz and Illmensee (1975) reported that malignant mouse teratocarcinoma cells which were taken from ascites tumors, grown in culture for 8 years and then injected into mouse blastocysts give rise to animals of normal appearance. The presence of genetic markers of the teratocarcinoma cells was unequivocally demonstrated in various tissues of the animals. These results strongly suggest that the event leading to the teratocarcinoma was not a genetic alteration, but it also may be that expression of genetically determined malignancy is dependent on certain cytoplasmic environmental factors which are not present in blastocysts. In fact, the strong regulatory effect of the cytoplasm on the expression of malignancy has been clearly demonstrated by Howell and Sager (1978). In reciprocal fusions between malignant and nonmalignant cell lines from mouse and Chinese hamster, they demonstrated that malignancy was suppressed in some cytoplasmic backgrounds, partially suppressed in others and not suppressed in still others. They concluded that malignancy is probably determined genetically and that its expression may be modified by cytoplasmic factors.

In summary, most data favour a genetic event (gene mutation?) as the primordial cause of cancer induction through chemicals and other data suggest that the phenotypic expression (malignancy) of this mutation is under control of cytoplasmic constituents (see also Fidler, 1978).

4. DETECTION OF MUTAGENS AND THE IMPORTANCE OF COMPARATIVE TESTING

Another way of investigating the possible correlation between mutation and cancer induction by chemicals is comparative testing of a series of known carcinogens and noncarcinogens in a variety of test systems. Ideally the tests should be performed in the same animal (in order to eliminate differences in pharmacokinetics and metabolism) but this is not yet possible on a large scale. One principal reason is that there is a shortage of appropriate somatic mutation tests in, for instance, several organs of rodents. There are some promising methods under development in specific organs (Dean and Senner, 1977; Fahrig, 1977; Strauss and Albertini, 1977) but at present the most useful data for comparison have been obtained using lower organisms (mutagenicity test systems overview: see Mohn, 1978).

The quantitative aspect of the correlation varied very much with the state of development of the mutation detection systems. After the first successful demonstration of the mutagenic effects in Drosophila melanogaster of chemical carcinogens such as sulfur and nitrogen mustards by Auerbach and Robson (1944), several bacterial mutation systems were developed and have proven to be useful indicators of carcinogenic compounds (Witkin, 1947; Demerec, 1943, 1946; Kaplan, 1949, Iyer and Szybalski, 1958). But, then, reputed carcinogens such as benzidine, 2-naphthylamine, dialkylnitrosamines failed to be detected as mutagens in bacterial assays which were considered as of only minor usefulness for carcinogenicity testing. It was only after the recognition that many carcinogens exert their effects only after mammalian biotransformation to ultimately electrophilic reactants (see, for example, Miller, 1978), that mutagenicity test systems were developed which made use of the bacterial indicators as quick and reliable genetic systems and included representative parts of mammalian metabolism. Examples are the host-mediated assay (Gabridge et al., 1969) and the microsomal assay (Malling, 1971) in which cycasin and dialkylnitrosamines show mutagenic activity. Especially microsomal tests with bacteria have been further developed because of the availability of different genetic systems detecting most classes of gene mutations (see Kilbey et al., 1977), and among them, a test using Salmonella auxotrophs as genetic indicators was constructed by Ames et al. (1975) which is now in very wide use. This test was employed in a large scale comparative study involving 300 chemicals (McCann et al., 1975; McCann et al. 1976) which showed a high, but not absolute, correlation between mutagenicity and carcinogenicity, i.e., around 90% of the carcinogens tested are mutagenic in this "Ames-test" and only a few carcinogens are not mutagenic and a few non-carcinogens mutagenic. These results and the results obtained in another organism where a large number of substances have been tested, namely Drosophila melanogaster (Vogel and Sobels, 1976), strongly suggest a common target, i.e. a chromosomal gene(s), for both mutation and cancer induction. There are, however, notable exceptions of compounds which are carcinogenic in experimental animals but barely or not mutagenic, as depicted earlier in the text. Reason for the inability of detecting these chemicals as mutagens may lie in differences of metabolism of the test systems employed but also in the selective response of certain genes to given chemical mutagens. It must also be noted that the list of 300 chemicals used for comparison in the Ames-test may not have been completely representative of the actual situation: subsequent studies by Andrews et al. (1978a, 1978b) using nitrosamines and polynuclear hydrocarbons of known carcinogenic potency showed a reduced correlation of 80% and 58% for the nitrosamines and the polycyclic compounds, respectively. The correlation is further weakened by the fact that the Ames-test obviously needs further calibration and standardization, as demonstrated by different results with the same compound (SQ 18506) in different laboratories (Shahin and von Borstel, 1978; Sugimura et al., 1977), and by large differences in mutagenic response upon small variations of the testing procedure, e.g. in the case of co-mutagenic activity of nor-harman (Levitt et al., 1977; Nagao et al., 1977, 1978) and of other compounds (see Ashby and Styles, 1978a). These problems of calibration and standardization are now recognized and several comparative studies have been initiated using different genetic systems.

Taken together, it can be stated that comparative testing has empirically shown a high degree of correlation between mutagenicity and carcinogenicity of chemicals. The tests have not, however, demonstrated a causal relationship since the postulated common metabolites may react with different target molecules; furthermore, there are some indications that the metabolites (of the carcinogen N-hydroxy-N-2-fluorenylacetamide) ultimately responsible for malignancy are different from those which are mutagenically active in the Ames-test (Weeks et al., 1978). With regard to a possible quantitative correlation between carcinogenic potency in animals and mutagenic potency in bacterial systems, serious problems arise; most result from extreme differences in metabolism and pharmakokinetics in the different systems employed, especially if only microsomal preparations are used as representative of mammalian metabolism in mutagenicity tests. With certain classes of substances, such as the aflatoxins, there seems to be a partial quantitative correlation between carcinogenicity and mutagenic activity in several organisms (Wong et al., 1976; Callen et al., 1977) but a generalization seems premature and the current discussion which is actively processing (Ashby and Styles, 1978a; Ames and Hooper, 1978; Ashby and Styles, 1978b) only reiterates the need for further studies in this field. Especially, accurate measurement of dose to the DNA (the so-called molecular dosimetry) such as currently performed in a variety of organisms with the alkylating compound ethyl methane sulfonate (Aaron et al., 1978) will be a prerequisite for comparison of absolute efficiency of mutation and cancer induction. Furthermore, for several reasons which are depicted in a preliminary systematical study by Hussain and Ehrenberg (1977), back mutation systems will be of only restricted use for quantifying genetic effects inferred in the whole genome, and forward mutation detecting systems, ideally involving a multitude of genes, have to be further developed and calibrated in priority.

5. CONCLUSION

The recognition, through epidemiological studies, that environmental factors including chemicals and nutrition are of major importance in the etiology of cancer renders rapid and reliable detection of potential carcinogens necessary. The use of mutagenicity tests for this detection purpose is an attractive possibility since tests for mutagenicity have been developed in a wide variety of organisms (for overview, see Mohn, 1978) which allow the detection of many types of genetic alterations in a reasonably short period of time. In fact, comparative studies involving a large number of carcinogenic and noncarcinogenic chemicals have shown a high degree of qualitative correlation between mutagenicity and carcinogenicity. A question remains, however, if there is a causal relationship between the two phenomena (mutation and cancer initiation) and especially if the mutagenic potency of a given chemical is representative of its carcinogenic potency.

Arguments for and against such a causal relationship have been presented and evaluated and it appears that most data are indicative of a genetic alteration (gene mutation?) in the DNA as the causative event; especially the stochastic properties of the two phenomena and the fact that the kinds of compounds which cause each effect are in many cases the same on a qualitative basis argue strongly in favor of the mutational theory of at least certain cancer initiation processes. In view of these considerations, the use of mutagenicity tests for detecting carcinogens present in the environment seems appropriate and many of these tests are undergoing validation in a variety of laboratories. Studies are, furthermore, beginning to extend these qualitative data to a more quantitative and therefore predictive capacity.

ACKNOWLEDGEMENTS

The author is very thankful to Professor Dr. F.H. Sobels and to Dr. Charles S. Aaron for comments and for critically reading the manuscript.

REFERENCES

Aaron, C.S., A.A. Van Zeeland, G.R. Mohn and A.T. Natarajan (1978). Molecular dosimetry of the chemical mutagen ethyl methane sulfonate in Escherichia coli and in V-79 Chinese hamster cells. Mutation Res. 50: 419-426.
Ames, B.N. and K. Hooper (1978). Does carcinogenic potency correlate with mutagenic potency in the Ames assay? Nature 274: 19-20.
Ames, B.N., J. McCann and E. Yamasaki (1975). Methods for detecting carcinogens and mutagens with the Salmonella/mammalian-microsome mutagenicity test. Mutation Res. 31: 347-364.
Andrews, A.W., L.H. Thibault and W. Lijinsky (1978). The relationship between carcinogenicity and mutagenicity of some polynuclear hydrocarbons. Mutation Res. 51: 311-318.
Andrews, A.W., L.H. Thibault and W. Lijinsky (1978). The relationship between mutagenicity and carcinogenicity of some nitrosamines. Mutation Res. 51: 319-326.
Ashby, J. and J.A. Styles (1978a). Comutagenicity, competitive enzyme substrates, and in vitro carcinogenicity assays. Mutation Res. 54: 105-112.
Ashby, J. and J.A. Styles (1978b). Factors influencing mutagenic potency in vitro. Nature 274: 20-22.
Auerbach, C. (1976). Mutation Research. Problems, results and perspectives. Chapman and Hall, London, pp. 378-405.
Auerbach, C. and J.M. Robson (1944). Production of mutations by allyl isothiocyanate. Nature 154: 81-82.
Barrett, J.C. and P.O. Ts'O (1978). Relationship between somatic mutation and neoplastic transformation. Proc. Natl. Acad. Sci. 75: 3297-3301.
Barrett, J.C., T. Tsuitsui and P.O.P. Ts'o (1978). Neoplastic transformation induced by a direct perturbation of DNA. Nature 274: 229-232.
Bauer, K.H. (1928). Mutationstheorie der Geschwulstentstehung, Springer, Berlin.
Bell, J. (1876) Edinb. Med. J. 22: 135.
Blot, W.J., T.J. Mason, R. Hoover and J.F. Fraumeni (1977). Cancer by county. Etiological implications. In "Origins of Human Cancer", H.H. Hiatt, ed., Cold Spring Harb., pp. 21-32.
Bentvelzen, P. chapter 4, this volume.
Callen, D.F., G.R. Mohn and T.M. Ong (1977). Comparison of the genetic effects of Aflatoxins B1 and G1 in Escherichia coli and Saccharomyces cerevisiae. Mutation Res. 45: 7-11.
Clayson, D.B. (1962). Chemical carcinogenesis. Little Brown and Co., Boston.
Cleaver, J.E. (1975). Xeroderma pigmentosum, DNA repair and carcinogenesis. In "Cancer Genetics", H.T. Lynch, ed., C.C. Thomas, Springfield, pp. 111-121.
Dean, D.F. and K.R. Senner (1977). Detection of chemically-induced mutations in tissues of Chinese hamsters. In "Progress in Genetic Toxicology", D. Scott et al., eds., Elsevier/North Holland, pp. 201-206.
De Grouchy, J. and C. Turleau (1974). Clonal evolution in the myeloid leukemias. In "Chromosome and cancer", J. German, ed., John Wiley and Sons, London, pp. 287-311.
Demerec, M. (1946). Induced mutations and possible mechanisms of the transmission of heredity in Escherichia coli. Proc. Natl. Acad. Sci. 32: 36-46.
De-Thé, G., A. Geser, N.E. Day, P.M. Tukei, E.H. Williams, D.P. Beri, P.G. Smith, A.G. Dean, G.W. Bornkamm, P. Peorino and W. Henle (1978). Epidemiological evidence for causal relationship between Epstein-Barr virus and Burkitt's lymphoma from Ugandan prospective study. Nature 274: 756-761.
Dunn, J.E. (1975). Cancer epidemiology in populations of the United States −

with emphasis on Hawaii and California – and Japan. Cancer Res. 35: 3240-3245.

Van der Eb, A.J., chapter 5, this volume.

Fahrig, R. (1977). The mammalian spot test (Fellfleckentest) with mice. Arch. Toxicol. 38: 87-98.

Fialkow, P.J. (1977). Clonal origin and stem cell evolution of human tumors. In "Genetics of human cancer", J. Mulvihill et al., eds., Raven Press, New York, pp. 439-453.

Fidler, I.J. (1978). Tumor heterogeneity and the biology of cancer invasion and metastasis. Cancer Res. 38: 2651-2660.

Gabridge, M.G. and M.S. Legator (1969). A host-mediated microbial assay for the detection of mutagenic compounds. Proc. Soc. Exptl. Med. Biol. 130: 831-834.

Gartler, S.M. (1974). Utilization of mosaic systems in the study of the origin and progression of tumors. In "Chromosome and cancer", J. German, ed., John Wiley and Sons, New York, pp. 313-334.

German, J. (1974). Chromosomes and cancer, John Wiley and Sons, New York.

Glickman, B.W., chapter 3, this volume.

Hart, R.W., Setlow, R.B. and A.D. Woodhead (1977). Evidence that pyrimidine dimers can give rise to tumors. Proc. Natl. Acad. Sci. 74: 5574-5578.

Hiatt, H.H., J.D. Watson, J.A. Winsten, eds. (1977). Origins of human cancer, Cold Spring Harbor Conf. Cell Proliferation, Vol. 4, Book A, B, and C, Cold Spring Harbor Laboratory.

Higginson, J. (1969). Present trends in cancer epidemiology. Canadian Cancer Conf. 8: 40-76.

Hormozdiari, H., N.E. Day, B. Aramesh and E. Mahboubi (1975). Dietary factors and oesophageal cancer in the Caspian littoral of Iran. Cancer Res. 35: 3493-3498.

Howell, A.N. and R. Sager (1978). Tumorigenicity and its suppression in hybrids of mouse and Chinese hamster cell lines. Proc. Natl. Acad. Sci. 75: 2358-2362.

Hussain, S. and L. Ehrenberg (1977). Gene mutations: Dose-response relationships and their significance for extrapolation to man. Abhandl. Akad. Wissenschaften der DDR N9: 95-100.

IARC Monographs on the Evaluation of the Carcinogenic Risk of Chemicals to Humans. Vol. 1-18 (1972-1978), IARC, Lyon.

Iyer, V.N. and W. Szybalski (1958). Two simple methods for the detection of chemical mutagens. Appl. Microbiol. 6: 23-29.

Janerick, D.T. and C.F. Lawrence (1975). Epidemiological strategies for identifying carcinogens. Mutation Res. 33: 55-63.

Kaplan, R.W. (1949). Mutations by photodynamic action of Bacterium prodigiosum. Nature 163: 573-574.

Kilbey, B.J., M. Legator, W. Nichols and C. Ramel, eds. (1977). Handbook of Mutagenicity Test Procedures, Elsevier, Amsterdam.

Levitt, R.C. (1977). Effects of harman and nor-harman on the mutagenicity and binding to DNA of benzo(a)pyrene metabolites in vitro and on aryl hydrocarbon hydroxylase induction in cell culture. Biochem. Biophys. Res. Commun. 79: 1167-1175.

Loveless, A. (1969). Possible relevance of O^6-alkylation of deoxyguanosine to the mutagenicity and carcinogenicity of nitrosamines and nitrosamides. Nature 223: 206-207.

Lynch, H.T., ed. (1976). Cancer Genetics, C.C. Thomas, Springfield.

Magee, P.N. and J.M. Barnes (1967). Carcinogenic N-nitroso compounds, Adv. in Cancer Research 10: 163-246.

Malling, H.V. (1971). Dimethylnitrosamine: Formation of mutagenic compounds by interaction with mouse liver microsomes. Mutation Res. 13: 425-429.

McCann, J., E. Choi, E. Yamasaki and B.N. Ames (1975). Detection of carcinogens as mutagens in the Salmonella/microsome test: Assay of 300 chemicals. Proc. Natl. Acad. Sci. 72: 5135-5139.

McCann, J. and B.N. Ames (1976). Detection of carcinogens as mutagens in the Salmonella/microsome test: Assay of 300 chemicals. Discussion. Proc. Natl. Acad. Sci. 73: 950-954.

McKinnel, R.G., B.A. Deggins and D.D. Labat (1969). Transplantation of pluripotential nuclei from triploid frog tumors. Sciences 165: 394-395.

Miller, E.C. (1978). Some current perspectives on chemical carcinogenesis in humans and experimental animals. Presidential address. Cancer Res. 38: 1479-1496.

Mintz, B. and K. Illmensee (1975). Normal genetically mosaic mice produced from malignant teratocarcinoma cells. Proc. Natl. Acad. Sci. 72: 3585-3589.

Mishra, N.K., K.J. Pant, C.M. Wilson and F.O. Thomas (1977). Carcinogen-induced mutations at two separate genetic loci are not enhanced by leukemia virus infection. Nature 266: 548-550.

Mohn, G.R. (1978). An overview of animal and microbial test systems for carcinogenesis and mutagenesis. Problems with human variation. Human Genetics, Suppl. 1, pp. 169-176.

Montesano, R., H. Bartsch, L. Tomatis and W. Davis, eds. (1976). Screening tests in chemical carcinogenesis, IARC Scientific Publications No. 12, IARC, Lyon.

Montesano, R., L. Tomatis and W. Davis, eds. (1974). Chemical carcinogenesis assays, IARC Scientific Publication No. 10, IARC, Lyon.

Mulvihill, J.J., R.W. Miller and J. Fraumeni, eds. (1977). Genetics of Human Cancer, Raven Press, New York.

Nagao, M., T. Yahagi, T. Kawachi Y. Seino, M. Honda, N. Matsukara, T. Sugimura, K. Wakabayashi, K. Tsuji and T. Kosuge (1977). In "Progress in Genetic Toxicology", D. Scott et al., eds., Elsevier/North-Holland, Amsterdam, pp. 259-264.

Nagao, M., T. Yahagi and T. Sugimura (1978). Differences in effects of norharman with various classes of chemical mutagens and amounts of S-9 Biochem. Biophys. Res. Commun. 83: 373-378.

Nowell, P.C. (1974). Chromosome changes and the clonal evolution of cancer. In "Chromosome and Cancer", J. German, ed. John Wiley and Sons, New York, pp. 267-285.

Parodi, S. and G. Brambilla (1977). Relationships between mutation and transformation frequencies in mammalian cells treated "in vitro" with chemical carcinogens. Mutation Res. 47: 53-74.

Rajewsky, M.F. and R. Goth (1976). Nervous-system specificity of carcinogenesis by N-ethyl-N-nitrosourea in the rat/Possible significance of 0^6-guanine alkylation and DNA repair. In "Screening Tests in Chemical Carcinogenesis", R. Montesano et al., eds., IARC, Lyon, pp. 593-597.

Rehn, L. (1895). Blasengeschwülste bei Fuchsin-Arbeitern. Arch. Klin. Chir. 50: 588-600.

Reznikoff, C.A., J.S. Bertram, D.W. Brankow and C. Heidelberger (1973). Quantitative and qualitative studies of chemical transformation of cloned C3H mouse embryo cells sensitive to postconfluence inhibition of cell division. Cancer Res. 33: 3239-3249.

Shahin, M. and R.C. von Borstel (1978). Comparisons of mutation induction in reversion systems of Saccharomyces cerevisiae and Salmonella typhimurium. Mutation Res. 53: 1-10.

Singer, B. (1976). All oxygens in nucleic acids react with carcinogenic ethylating agents. Nature 264: 333-339.

Strauss, G.H. and R.J. Albertini (1977). 6-Thioguanine resistant lymphocytes in human peripheral blood. In "Progress in Genetic Toxicology", D. Scott et al., eds., Elsevier/North-Holland, Amsterdam, pp. 327-334.

Sugimura, T., T. Kawachi, T. Matsushima, M. Nagao, S. Sato and T. Yahagi (1977). A critical review of submammalian systems for mutagen detection. In "Progress in Genetic Toxicology", D. Scott et al., eds., Elsevier/North-Holland, Amsterdam, 125-140.

Thompson, L.H. and R.M. Baker (1973). Isolation of mutants in cultured mammalian cells. In "Methods in Cell Biology", D.M. Prescott, ed., Vol. VI, pp. 209-281.

Trosko, J.E. and E.H.Y. Chu (1975). The role of DNA repair and somatic mutation in carcinogenesis. Adv. Cancer Res. 21: 391-425.

Vogel, E. and F.H. Sobels (1976). The function of Drosophila in genetic toxicology testing. In "Chemical Mutagens. Principles and Methods for their Detection", A. Hollaender, ed., Vol. IV, Plenum Press, New York, pp. 93-142.

Volkmann, R. von (1875). Beiträge zur Chirurgie, Leipzig.

Wang, T., T. Kakizoe, P. Dion, R. Furrer, A.J. Varghese and W.R. Bruce (1978). Volatile nitrosamines in normal human faeces. Nature 276: 280-281.

Weeks, C.E., W.T. Allaben, S.C. Louie, E.J. Lazear and C.M. King (1978). Role of arylhydroxamic acid transferase in the mutagenicity of N-hydroxy-N-2-fluorenylacetamide in Salmonella typhimurium. Cancer Res. 38: 613-618.

Witkin, E.M (1947). Mutations in Escherichia coli induced by chemical agents. Cold Spring Harbor Symp. Quant. Biol. 12: 256-269.

Wogan, G.N. (1975). Dietary factors and special epidemiological situations of liver cancer in Thailand and Africa. Cancer Res. 35: 3499-3502.

Wolf, U. (1974). Theodor Boveri and his book "On the problem of the origin of malignant tumors". In "Chromosomes and Cancer", J. German, ed., John Wiley and Sons, New York, pp. 3-20.

Wong, J.J. and D.P.H. Hsieh (1976). Mutagenicity of aflatoxins related to their metabolism and carcinogenic potential. Proc. Natl. Acad. Sci. 73: 2241-2244.

Wynder, E.L. and G.B. Gori (1977). Contribution of the environment to cancer incidence: An epidemiological exercise. J. Nath. Cancer Inst. 58: 825-832.

Yamagiwa, K. and K. Ichikawa (1915). Mult. med. Fak. Tokio 15: 295.

3. DNA REPAIR AND ITS RELATIONSHIP TO THE ORIGINS OF HUMAN CANCER

BARRY W. GLICKMAN

ABSTRACT

The existence of certain repair deficient human disorders and the associated prevalence of cancer among affected individuals provides clues to how potentially dangerous environmental agents which are capable of causing alterations in the structure of DNA may result in human cancer. Here evidence is reviewed concerning the somatic mutation theory of the origin of cancer and the influence of known DNA repair processes on both mutagenesis and cancer is considered.

The past several years both laymen and scientists have been paying increased attention to the role of environmental factors in relation to the occurrence of human cancers. This increased interest stems from an influx of evidence that the majority of human cancers are the result of environmental agents which ultimately react with and damage our DNA. Four major sources of evidence have contributed to the opinion that cancer is the result of environmental factors which damage the DNA: (1) epidemiological evidence, (2) the high degree of correlation between mutagens and potential carcinogens, (3) the induction of cancer by UV-light DNA photoproducts and (4) the relationship between DNA repair and cancer as evidenced by a persistence of DNA damage in tissues most sensitive to a given carcinogen and the prevalence of cancer in humans having a defect in the repair of DNA damage.

1. EPIDEMIOLOGICAL EVIDENCE

The involvement of environmental factors in carcinogenesis is based in part on the conclusions of epidemiologists such as Higginson (1969) and Blot et al. (1977) who, on the basis of the differences in the occurrence of cancer in different geographic locations, estimated that 60-90% of all human cancer was strongly influenced by an important

F.J. Cleton and J.W.I.M. Simons (eds.), Genetic Origins of Tumor Cells. 25–51.
Copyright © 1980 by Martinus Nijhoff Publishers bv, The Hague/Boston/London.
All rights reserved.

environmental factor. This deduction was further supported by Haenzsel and his collaborators (1968, 1973, 1975), who showed that these differences were not primarily genetically determined.

2. CORRELATION BETWEEN MUTAGENS AND CARCINOGENS

Interest in this area has been further intensified by the finding that 75-90% of all carcinogens are mutagens (McCann et al., 1975a, 1975b; Bridges, 1976). This aspect of the origins of human cancer is more fully discussed in the review by G. Mohn in this volume.

3. CANCER AS A RESULT OF UV-INDUCED DNA DAMAGE

There has been strong circumstantial evidence for the involvement of DNA damage in the induction of skin cancer by "natural" ultra-violet light (Emmett, 1973; Urbach et al., 1972) but direct evidence for the involvement of UV damage has been lacking. Direct evidence for the involvement of UV-induced DNA damage in the induction of cancer has been obtained by Hart and Setlow (1975), who took advantage of some unusual characteristics of the Amazon molly (*Poecelia formosa*) which reproduces asexually so that the offspring of one female constitute a clone. As a result, tissue can be transplanted from one individual to another without immunological barriers. Moreover, the major UV-induced damage, pyrimidine dimers (see Figure 1) can be efficiently photoreactivated in the tissues of the fish (see Figure 2 for a summary of the error-free DNA repair pathways). These characteristics of *Poecelia formosa*

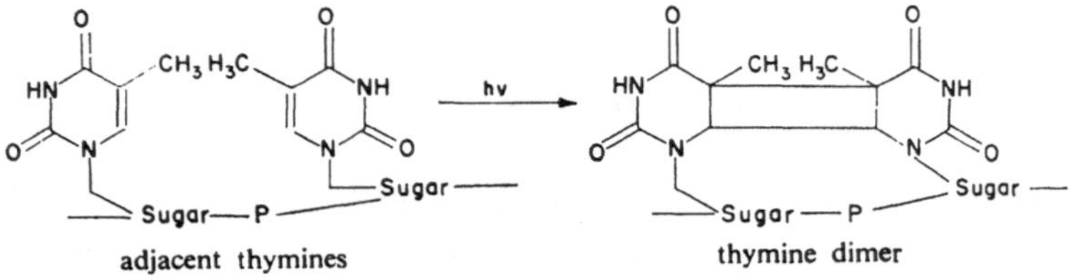

adjacent thymines   thymine dimer

Figure 1. The pyrimidine dimer. The major DNA photoproduct of UV-light is the cyclobutane pyrimidine dimer formed between adjacent pyrimidine in the same strand. The illustration shows the formation of a thymine dimer.

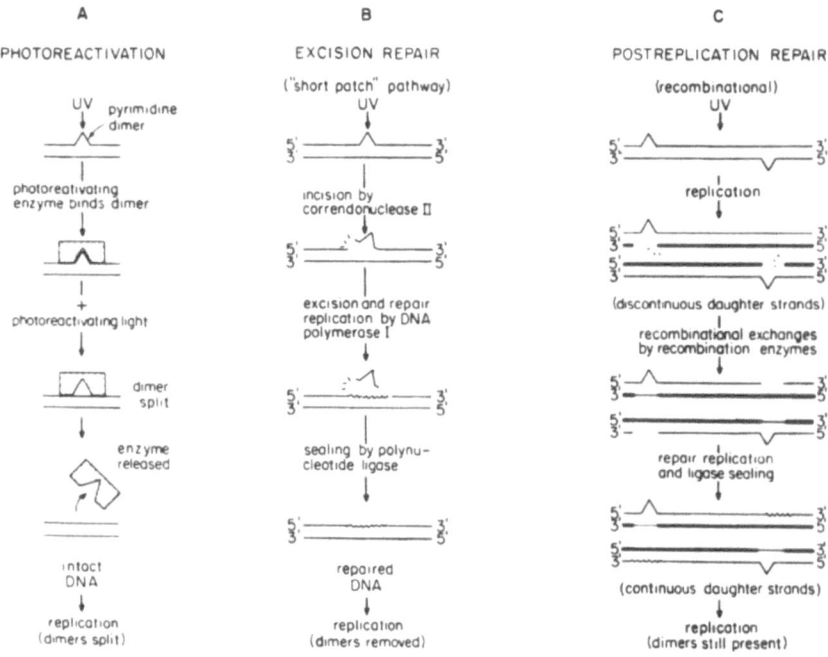

Figure 2. The "Error-free" pathways of the enzymatic repair of DNA damage as caused by UV-light in *Escherichia coli* (from Witkin, 1976). Photoreactivation (A) involves the in situ reversion of the dimers by the photoreactivating enzyme and visible light. Excison repair (B) is the enzymatically directed specific removal of the pyrimidine dimer. This process involves the recognition of the damage; incision at or near the damaged site; the enzymatic removal of the dimer; resynthesis of the excised region and ligation to restore the continuity of the DNA molecule. Postreplication Repair (C) differs from the first two modes of DNA repair in that rather than resulting in the removal of the damage, postreplication repair permits the cell to "tolerate" the lesion. Postreplication repair is a complex process involving at least five pathways (Kimball, 1978). Symbols: ‾V‾ or _∧_ denote a pyrimidine dimer; the heavy lines are the DNA daughter strands produced by the first post-irradiation replication; the light lines are the original UV-irradiated parental strands; the wavy lines show strands synthesized during repair replication.

enabled Hart and Setlow to show not only that cells UV-irradiated in vitro cause tumours upon transplantation but that, if the irradiated cells were first subjected to photoreactivation, the tumorigenic effect was reversed. This provides strong evidence that the DNA lesion, in this case the pyrimidine dimer, was responsible for the initiation of tumorigenesis.

4. PERSISTENCE OF LESIONS IN THE DNA AND SUSCEPTIBILITY TO TUMORIGENESIS

In early studies, the observation that alkylating agents were inactivating to the DNA (Herriot, 1948) and mutagenic (Auerbach and Robson, 1947) was correlated with the level of N^7-alkylguanine in the DNA (Singer, 1975). While N^7-alkylguanine was presumed to be of biological significance, its presence did not change base pairing specificity (Ludlum, 1970; Gerchman and Ludlum, 1973) and its effects were attributed to rapid depurination and chain breakage. However, when highly carcinogenic N-nitroso compounds were used to modify nucleic acid in vitro or in vivo another derivative, O^6-alkylguanine, was found which represented a few percent of the total alkyl groups (Lawley et al., 1970, 1972a, b; Walker and Ewart, 1973; Kleihues and Magee, 1973; Goth and Rajewsky, 1974; Singer and Frankel-Conrat, 1975). When the reaction was performed with agents of low carcinogenicity, this derivative was not detected or was present in only trace amounts (Lawley et al., 1970, 1972a; Walker and Ewart, 1973; Singer and Frankel-Conrat, 1975; Sun and Singer, 1975; Craddock, 1973). Not only was a correlation established between carcinogenicity and the persistence of 6-alkylguanine but 6-alkylguanine has been shown to mispair (Gerchman and Ludlum, 1975; Abdulner and Flurry, 1976) and can thus be considered mutagenic. Moreover, the specific removal of 6-alkylguanine from DNA has been demonstrated in mammalian cells (Kirtikar and Goldthwait, 1974; Singer 1976; Goth and Rajewsky, 1974) and in rats given N-methyl-N-nitrosourea (MNUA) or N-ethyl-N-nitrosourea (ENUA) under conditions where only brain tumours develop, excision occurs much more slowly from nervous tissue than any of the non-tumour producing tissues examined (Goth and Rajewsky, 1974; Margison and Kleihues, 1975; Kleihues and Margison, 1974, 1976; Rajewsky et al., 1976). Similarly, the persistence of 6-alkylguanine in kidney cells compared with liver cells following treatment with dimethyl-nitrosamines has been correlated with tumour forming in the kidney (Nicoll et al., 1975).

The persistence of mispairing and therefore mutagenic lesions in tissues most susceptible to tumour induction by the specific alkylating agent provides a further indication that DNA damage and mutagenesis are in some way related to tumour induction.

5. REPAIR DEFICIENCY AND HUMAN CANCER

While a growing body of evidence exists suggesting a causal relationship between DNA damage, mutagenesis and tumour induction, the best evidence that human cancer can arise as a consequence of DNA damage comes from the observation that several human disorders which result in a defect in the cell's ability to repair certain chemical and physical lesions in the DNA are also associated with increased frequencies of cancer among affected individuals (German, 1972; Setlow, 1978). Three such diseases are xeroderma pigmentosum (XP), ataxia telangiectasia (AT) and Fanconi's anemia (FA).

5.1. Xeroderma pigmentosum

XP is an autosomal, recessively inherited skin disease in which the homozygotes show a marked tendency to develop skin cancer upon exposure to sunlight. Since the discovery by Cleaver (1968) that cells from XP homozygotes are defective in the reinsertion of new bases into the DNA of UV irradiated cells, a process referred to as unscheduled DNA synthesis (UDS), XP has become the most widely studied human repair deficiency (see reviews by Cleaver and Bootsma, 1975; Cleaver, 1978).

While all XP individuals are defective in at least one mode of DNA repair of UV light induced damage, most XP individuals show a defect in excision repair (see Figure 2). The extent of this defect varies from greater than 90% in some individuals to only 50% in others (see Table 1). Cells taken from affected individuals are UV sensitive (Cleaver, 1970; Goldstein, 1971; Takebe et al., 1972; Stich et al., 1973) and have a reduced capacity to reactivate UV irradiated viruses such as SV40 (Aaronson and Lytle, 1970), vaccinia (Zádová, 1971; Lytle et al., 1972), herpes simplex virus (Lytle et al., 1972; Rabson et al., 1969) and adenovirus (Day, 1974a, b). The rate of the removal of UV-induced pyrimidine dimers (Figure 1) is greatly reduced in XP cells (Setlow et al., 1969; Cleaver and Trosko, 1970) as is the rate of the disappearance of UV-endonuclease sensitive sites (Paterson et al., 1973).

5.1.1. Genetic analysis
Genetic analysis of defective DNA repair in XP cells can be carried out by cell fusion procedures. By this technique, hybrid, multinucleate cells (heterokaryons) are exposed to UV light and the level of unscheduled DNA synthesis (UDS) is measured. Using this technique, Kraemer et al. (1975) originally

Table 1. DNA repair properties and general characteristics of different classes of XP.

XP class [1]	% DNA repair [2]	% Photo-reactivation [3]	Excision in vivo after T4 UV endo [4]	Incision in vitro without freezing [5]	Excision in vitro after freezing [6]	Activity of apurinic endonuclease [7]
A	2-5%	0-36%	+	+	+	altered K_m
B	3-7%	0%	+	−	−	+
C	5-20%	15.8%	+	+	+	+
D	25-50%	8%	+	+	+	15-20% normal altered K_m
E	40-50%	50%	+	−	+	+
F	10%	?	?	?	?	?
G	?	?	?	?	?	?
Variants	100%	5-50%	n.a.	n.a.	n.a.	?

[1] General XP symptoms include hypersensitivity of the skin to sunlight, dry atrophic skin, excessive keratosis and freckling. Cancers may develop to varying degrees in different patients depending upon genetic make up and exposure to sunlight (Robbins et al., 1974). [2] Given as percent UDS relative to normal cells (Cleaver and Bootsma, 1975). [3] Given as percent photoreactivation compared to normal cells (Sutherland, 1975, 1977). [4] Based upon the results of Tanaka et al. (1975) using Sendai virus permeabilized cells and T4 UV-endonuclease. [5] Incision measured using purified *E. coli* DNA irradiated with UV: Data of Mortelman et al. (1976) and Cook et al. (1975). [6] Based upon data of Friedberg et al. (1974). [7] Based upon data of Kuhnlein et al. (1976, 1978).

described five complementation groups, A through E. More recently two new groups, F (Takebe, 1978) and G (Bootsma, 1978) have been described.

5.1.2. XP variants A second general class of XP deficiency also exists, the XP-variants in which the affected individuals share some common clinical features, but whose cells show no reduction of UDS following UV irradiation and only slightly increased sensitivity to the lethal effects of UV (Cleaver, 1972). Lehman et al. (1975) have shown XP-varients to be defective in post replication repair and its associated gap closure (see Figure 2). Moreover, caffeine, known to disturb post replication repair, sensitizes the XP variant cells to UV but not normal cells (Lehman et al., 1975).

5.1.3. Biochemical defect The biochemical characterization of XP cells has led to a number of observations showing enormous heterogeneity suggesting that XP's include a number of genetic defects, all of which adversely affect DNA repair. The XP groups and their general characteristics are summarized in Table 1. The picture has emerged, at least for most XP cases, that the XP defect affected the initial step in DNA repair, the incision step (Cleaver, 1969; Setlow et al., 1969). Indeed, experiments by Tanaka et al. (1975) showed XP cells of groups A through E rendered permeable to purified T4 UV-specific endonuclease by Sendai virus treatment, to have normal repair. Moreover, Friedberg et al. (1974), taking advantage of the fact that after freezing and thawing the ability of human cell extracts to incise UV-irradiated DNA is lost, showed the XP groups, A, C, D and E capable of completing the excision repair process on UV-irradiated *E. coli* DNA pre-incised with T4 UV-endonuclease. This demonstrated that these XP groups had post-incision DNA repair steps. Mortelman and her colleagues (1976) have shown that unfrozen extracts of XP complementation groups A and C are capable of incision using purified UV-irradiated *E. coli* DNA in vitro. Cook et al. (1975) demonstrated similar activities in extracts from both group A and D XP cells. It is apparent therefore, that while XP cells are incapable of carrying out the incision step in vivo, certain groups are able to carry out this step in vitro. The situation is thus more complex than originally envisioned by Cleaver (1969) and Setlow et al. (1969). A partial explanation of the difference between the relatively simple excision system described by Grossman (1974) for prokaryotes and that seen in human cells may be related to differences in chromosomal organization. The DNA of eukaryotes is highly organized into repeating nucleosome structures consisting of core DNA (about 140 base pairs) associated with four pairs of histone molecules linked to the adjacent nucleosomes by an approximately 50 base pair length of linker DNA (Kornberg, 1977; Oudet et al., 1975). The observation that extracts of XP groups A, C and D can carry out the incision step on purified DNA in vitro suggests that the deficiency in vivo may involve a question of access to the chromosomal DNA so that the excision repair process in eukaryotes requires additional components not anticipated from work on prokaryotes, but may involve multi-functional-multi-enzyme systems as suggested by Haynes (1966).

5.1.4. XP and UV- induced mutagenesis The frequency of induction of 8-azaguanine-resistant mutants in XP cells by UV light is higher in XP fibroblasts than observed in normal cells (Maher and McCormick, 1975; Maher et al., 1976) in a manner reminiscent of *E. coli* strains defective in excision repair (Ishii and Kondo, 1975). As presented in Figure 2, cells possess a number of error-free repair processes which allow the efficient removal of DNA lesions and the restoration of viability while avoiding mutation. As will be discussed more fully later, alternative repair mechanisms exist which, while increasing cellular survival, do so at the cost of fidelity. The later repair pathways are referred to as "error-prone" while the accurate repair pathways are "error-free". As XP cells show an increase in mutagenesis, the defect in DNA repair is in an "error-free" pathway such that survival must be promoted by an error-prone DNA repair mechanism.

5.1.5. XP and the repair of DNA damage caused by chemical carcinogens Bacteria that are defective in excision repair are also defective in the repair of damage caused by a number of chemical agents and the same is true for XP cells. In general, XP cells are sensitive to agents which cause DNA adducts requiring excision repair of large patch size, involving 30-100 nucleotides (Regan and Setlow, 1974) while XP cells remain competent in the repair of X-ray "like" lesions involving single-strand break repair or lesions involving relatively short patches of DNA repair (Painter and Young, 1972). The repair capability of XP cells is summarized in Table 2.

Table 2. DNA damaging agents and/or their products and the repair ability of XP cells (Adopted from Setlow (1978), Cleaver (1978) and Cleaver and Bootsma (1975)). A listing in both categories means that an agent produces different products or that different cell lines have given a different result.

Repair deficient	Repair proficient
Ultraviolet (sunlight)	Ionising radiation
− dimers	− strand breaks
− protein DNA links	− anoxic
− strand breaks	4-NQO (minor comp)
Ionising radiation-anoxic (base damage)	
4-NQO	
AAF damage	Bromouracil photoproducts
ICR-170	
1-Nitropyridine-1-oxide	Mitomycin (bifunctional)
EMS (primarily mispairing)	EMS
O^6-alkylGua (mispairing)	MNNG
Psoralen + light (cross-links)	MNU
BCNU	
HNO_2	N^7 alkylGuanine (depurination and
Propane sultone	ss-breaks)
Decarbamyl mito C (monofunctional)	Proflavin + light
Acetylaminofluorene	
Aflatoxin	
K---region epoxides	
Br benzanthracene	
Br_2 Me benzanthracene	

5.1.6. The question of chromosomal structure and the problem of "access" As pointed out earlier, the eukaryotic chromosome is a highly organized structure presenting an "access" problem to the cell's repair enzymes. The same applies to the "access" of some chemical agents to the DNA as chemical carcinogens generally affect the linker, i.e. micrococcal, nuclease accessible region of the DNA (Moses et al., 1976; Ramanathan et al., 1976; Jahn and Litman, 1977; Metzger et al., 1977). Moreover, "access" also influences the rate at which alkylation damage resulting from the treatment in vivo of rat liver cells with dimethylnitrosamine disappears from the DNA (Ramanathon et al., 1976). An analysis by Cleaver (1977) showed dimers to be removed mor readily from linker DNA than core DNA. This is consistent with the data of Paterson et al. (1973) who found that there were two rates at which UV-endonuclease specific sites disappeared from UV-irradiated DNA.

From these results one might suggest that if a chemical agent is specific for linker DNA, those XP complementation groups defective in excision repair by virtue of problems of access would show better survival on exposure to such agents than XP cells defective in the actual excision process itself. At the present time, however, insufficient information is available to confirm or negate this hypothesis.

5.2. Ataxia telangiectasia

Ataxia telangiectasia (AT) is a progressive, multifaceted disorder having neurological, oculocutaneous and immunological complications (Sedgewick and Border, 1972; Kraemer, 1977). The present estimate is that 10% of AT homozygotes develop cancers at an early age. This is more than 100 times greater than the general population in age matched controls. The discovery that AT patients react severely to radiotherapy (Cunliffe et al., 1975) has stimulated research on the repair capacity of AT cells. Indeed, AT cells are about 3-5 times more sensitive to ionizing radiation than normal cells (Taylor et al., 1976) and show increased levels of both spontaneous and induced chromosomal aberration (Higurashi and Conen, 1973). While AT cells are able to repair both single and double strand breaks quite efficiently (Taylor, 1975; Lehman and Stevens, 1977), AT cells are more sensitive to MNNG and antinomycin D (Scudiero, 1978; Hoar and Sargeant, 1976). However, the situation with AT is less straightforward than with XP because no environmental agent is known to be responsible for the increased cancer frequency and, in contrast to the hypermutability of XP cells by UV, AT cells are *hypomutable* by X-

rays (Arlett, 1977). This means that either the X-ray lesions go
unrepaired and the damage is lethal or that an important component
for the repair of these lesions is error-prone and absent in AT cells.
Data from Paterson et al. (1976) showing that AT strains deficient in
X-ray induced repair replication are impaired in the removal of sites
sensitive to a damage specific endonuclease isolated from *Micrococcus
luteus* suggests that the lesions themselves are not mutagenic, but that
rather the defective repair process is error-prone. There are however,
many possible other interpretations for this result.

Heterozygotes for AT are moderately radiation sensitive (Lavin
et al., 1978; Paterson et al., 1978) and show a predisposition to
cancer; Swift (1976) estimates that 5% of all persons dying of cancer
before the age of 45 are likely to be AT heterozygotes. Since approximately 1% of the population is heterozygous for AT, the relative
importance of the exposure of such persons to ionizing radiation and
radiomimetic chemicals may represent a significant health problem.

5.3. Fanconi's anemia

The predominant clinical features of this complex syndrome are hema-
tological disturbances affecting all elements of the bone marrow com-
plicated by excessive bleeding and regular infections. Those who
survive childhood are prone to cancer, particularly leukemia and it
has been estimated (Swift, 1971) that 5% of all individuals dying of
leukemia are FA heterozygotes. Since the estimates for heterozygotes
in the general population is one in several hundreds, the increase in
proneness for the development of leukemia is significant.

While FA patients from a heterogeneous population, FA cells are
generally more sensitive to killing by mitomycin C than normal
cells (Higurashi and Coenen, 1973) as well as by psoralen and black
light (Sasaki and Tonomura, 1973). FA cells are also somewhat
sensitive to ionizing radiation and high doses of UV irradiation
(Rainbow and Howes, 1977; Poon et al., 1974). The DNA repair
defect in these cells appears to be involved in the repair of DNA cross-
links. However, in terms of mutability, FA cells behave like AT rather
than XP cells, i.e. they are hypomutable by mitomycin C, an agent
for which they are highly sensitive (Finkelberg et al., 1977).

Blood lymphocytes from affected individuals show a high
frequency of chromosomal aberrations including chromatid breaks
and gaps; rearrangements leading to dicentric chromosomes and
asymmetric quadriradials are not uncommon (German, 1972). Chromatid anomalies are increased above normal levels following treatment

of FA cells with agents such as mitomycin C to which the cells are sensitive (Sasaki and Tonomura, 1973). Interestingly, the level of sister chromatid exchanges (SCE's) in FA cells is normal (Kato and Stich, 1976) and even reduced following treatment by mitomycin C (Latt et al. 1975).

6. CELLULAR MECHANISMS OF MUTATION IN *E. COLI*

Mutagenesis in *E. coli* is thought to be primarily due to two major mechanisms: "indirect mutagenesis" provoked by noncoding, so called "bulky" lesions which inhibit DNA replication, and "direct mutagenesis" provoked by subtle modifications of the DNA template or incoming precursors. In the case of indirect mutagenesis, the noncoding lesions (e.g. pyrimidine dimers) obstruct DNA synthesis and result in the induction of the *recA* dependent SOS system (see Witkin, 1976 for a review) which at the cost of fidelity enables the cell to bypass the lesion (Radman, 1975; Radman et al., 1977; Villani et al., 1978).

Direct mutagenesis on the other hand can be due to tautomers and isomers of the normal bases (Watson and Crick, 1953; Topal and Fresco, 1976) or the incorporation of base analogues such as 2-aminopurine (2AP), 5-bromouracil (5BU) or 6-N-Hydroxylaminopurine (6-HAP) which successfully cheat the proof-reading 3'-5' error correcting activity of the bacterial repair system, deaminating agents such as bisulfite, hydroxylamine and nitrous acid or some alkylating agents (see Drake and Baltz, 1976, for a review). Direct mutagenesis is reflected in both spontaneous mutation and *recA* independent modes of mutagenesis (for a review, see Radman et al., 1978).

6.1. Indirect mutagenesis: The "SOS" DNA repair pathway

The question of the induction of the SOS pathway has been recently reviewed by Witkin (1976), Lehmann and Bridges (1977) and Kimball (1978). In short it suffices to say that DNA lesions blocking DNA replication initiate a series of events including the induction of protein X, the *recA* gene protein. The *recA* protein has proteolytic properties capable of inactivating the repressor protein of bacteriophage λ by cleaving it into two parts (Roberts et al., 1977; Roberts et al., 1978). It is suspected that the inactivation of certain suppressors by the *recA* gene product results in the activation of the SOS repair pathway. The cellular signals turning on SOS are still unknown. There is reason to

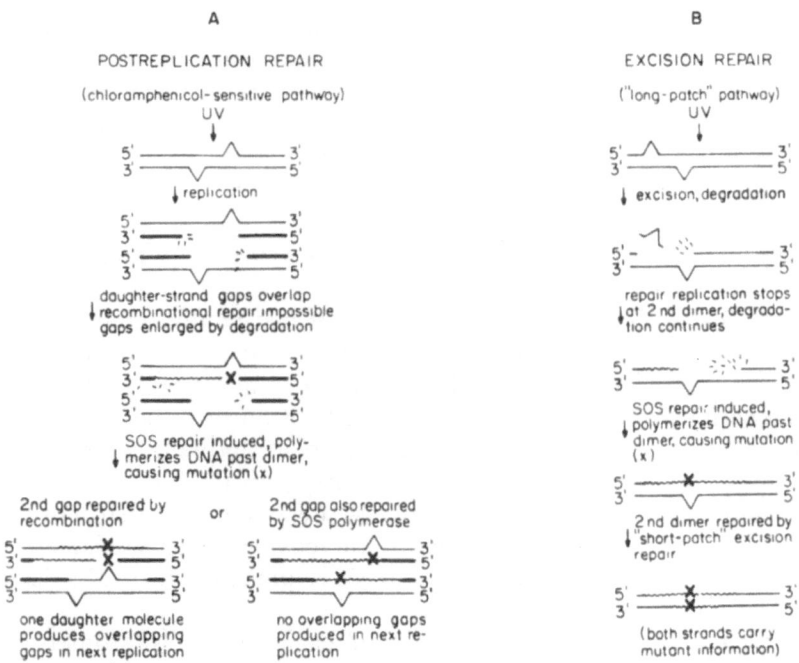

Figure 3. Possible pathways of "Error-prone" repair of damage caused by UV light (from Witkin, 1976). Two mechanisms are envisioned, one involving post-replication repair (A), the other excision repair (B). Both processes have in common however, that the presence of the pyrimidine dimer blocks DNA replication because such lesions are non-coding i.e. do not possess base pairing properties. At such sites DNA polymerase "idles" because its 3'-5' exonucleolytic activity effectively prevents replication past the dimer. It is thought that the induction of SOS repair permits replication past the dimer, possibly by the suppression of the proof-reading capacity of the polymerase (Witkin, 1976; Radman et al., 1977; Villani et al., 1978). The loss of proof-reading and synthesis over the non-coding dimer results in the errors which make this process error-prone. Symbols as in Figure 2; the site of the incorporation error and mutation is denoted by an X.

believe however, that the initial signals involve DNA breakdown products (Oishi et al., 1978) and/or blockage of DNA replication. The actual mechanism of SOS bypass may be related to the specific repression of the proof-reading functions of SOS (Figure 3 and Villani et al., 1978; Witkin, 1976). Villani et al. (1978) demonstrated in vitro the phenomenon of DNA polymerase "idling" on pyrimidine dimer containing ØX DNA template. Idling is the turnover of nucleoside triphosphate precursors to free nucleoside monophosphates in the absence of chain elongation. No new DNA polymerase or terminal transferase has been detected in extracts prepared from SOS "switched on" bacteria (Radman et al., 1977; Schaaper, Cohen and Glickman, unpublished observations). Moreover, DNA polymerase III seems to be involved in the SOS mutational process (Bridges et al., 1976). Evidence supporting the hypothesis that SOS related "bypass" repair might reflect reduced levels of the 3'-5' proof-reading exonuclease can be taken from the observation of "undirected mutagenesis" in cells where SOS has been switched on using the *tifA44* mutation which demonstrate all the SOS associated functions at 42° (Witkin, 1974, 1976) or a strain constitutive for SOS repair (Mount, 1977). In both these cases, increases in the spontaneous mutation rate suggest a lowering in DNA replication fidelity. Results from our laboratory (Schaaper and Glickman, unpublished) show terminal mismatch correction on artificial DNA template to be reduced in extracts made from "SOS" on *polA1* cells. While it is difficult to draw conclusions from experiments with crude extracts the exonucleolytic activity present in uninduced cells was NEM* sensitive and ATP independent, which would not be in contradiction with a role for the 3'-5' exonucleolytic activity of DNA polymerase III in this phenomenon. Results of Villani (1978) are consistent with these observations and support this model for SOS repair. Recent studies of bacteriophage T4 infected cells show error-prone repair to be abolished when T4-antimutator phages having an increased proof-reading capacity are used (Yarosh, 1978). This result provides in vivo support for the concept that the proof-reading function of DNA polymerase may play a vital role in mutation fixation following UV-irradiation.

6.2. SOS repair in mammalian cells?

The question of the involvement of inducible repair processes in mutagenesis in mammalian cells has become the concern of several laboratories. The pre-irradiation of mammalian cells leads to increased survival of UV-irradiated herpes virus (Bockstahler and Lytle, 1970, 1971) and adenovirus (Bockstahler, 1977). More recently Sarasin and Hanawalt (1978) demonstrated that the pretreatment of monkey kidney cells with carcinogens resulted in a protein synthesis dependent increase in the survival of UV-irradiated SV40 virus.

6.3. Mechanism of mammalian "bypass" repair

Purified mammalian DNA polymerases α, β and γ have been shown to

* NEM = N-ethyl-maleimide, an inhibitor of DNA polymerase III.

be devoid of exonuclease activity (Weisbach, 1977). Unlike bacterial polymerases, purified mammalian polymerases can efficiently copy pyrimidine dimer containing templates in vitro (Radman et al., 1977, 1978; Villani et al., 1978).

In vivo however, pyrimidine dimers do block DNA replication (Lehmann, 1972). The difference between in vitro and in vivo observations suggests that in vivo mammalian polymerases do operate in conjugation with a 3'-5' proof reading exonuclease. Indeed, the very high error rate (i.e. misincorporation level) of purified mammalian DNA polymerases compared to in vivo error rates may present further confirmatory evidence (Villani et al., 1978).

Recently, a 3'-5' exonucleolytic function has been partially purified from calf spleen (Spadari et al., personal communication; Radman et al., 1978). Interestingly, the re-addition of the purified exonuclease to purified calf spleen DNA polymerase α reduces the ability of the polymerase to synthesize on irradiated templates, strongly suggesting that the purified exonuclease can supply a proof-reading function.

In summary, the enzymatic machinery supplying a "bypass" mechanism for bulky lesions is present in mammalian cells. The question of whether SOS operates in mammalian cells and if it involves these enzymes remains to be seen.

6.4. Direct mutagenesis of E. coli

Spontaneous base alterations are estimated to occur in *E. coli* at the frequency of 10^{-10} errors per nucleotide per replication (Fowler et al., 1974). This remarkable fidelity can be accredited to (1) nucleotide discrimination by the DNA polymerase (the so-called "sticking time") between correct vs. incorrect nucleotide pairs, (2) the proof-reading, i.e. editing, function of the polymerase (see Radman et al., 1977; Brutlag and Kornberg, 1972; Gillin and Nosal, 1976) and (3) a post replicational error-avoidance mechanism which recognizes and corrects mismatched DNA in a directed manner (Glickman et al., 1978; Radman et al., 1978; Rykowski, Pukkila, Radman, Wagner and Meselson, personal communication).

7. ROLE FOR 6-METHYL ADENINE RESIDUES IN ERROR-AVOIDANCE

The occurrence of mismatch correction suggests that mismatch repair acts in a directed fashion to correct errors following DNA replication.

Inherent in such a mechanism is the requirement that the "correct" parental strand be distinguished from the "error containing" daughter strand. Wagner and Meselson (1976) suggested that the undermethylation of the newly replicated DNA strand might provide the basis for strand discrimination. Using bacteriophage λ heteroduplexes prepared from methylated and nonmethylated DNA, Rykowski et al. (1978) found that heteroduplex correction preferentially proceeded in the direction of the methylated strand. Thus, at mismatched sites, correction endonucleases generally chose the under-methylated DNA strand for correction, using the methylated strand preferentially as template.

E. coli mutants carrying the *dam* mutation are defective in methylation at 5'-G-A-T-C-3' sequence (Lacks and Greenberg, 1977) and are almost totally deficient in 6-methyladenine residues in their DNA (Marinus and Morris, 1974, 1975; Marinus, personal communication). The loss of DNA methylation results in increased spontaneous mutagenesis and hypermutability by base analogues (Glickman et al., 1978). These observations are consistent with the hypothesis that DNA methylation is involved in strand discrimination (see Figure 4). *Dam*

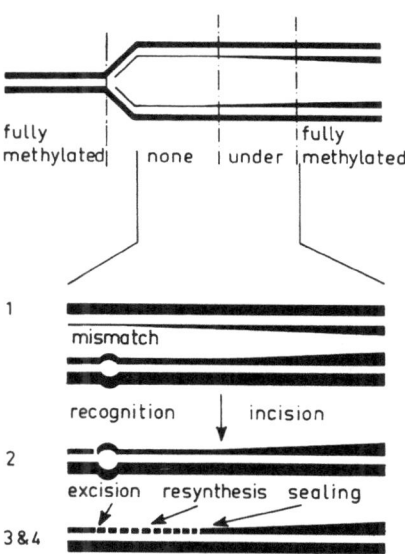

Figure 4. Model for methylation instructed error-avoidance. This post replicational error correcting system depends upon the under-methylation of the daughter strands following replication (thin lines) for strand discrimination during mismatch correction. The model involves (1) a DNA surveillance complex capable of recognizing a mismatched site and (2) performing the incision step at or near the site of the mismatch such that the daughter strand is cut. The mismatch is then excised (3); resynthesis and ligation follow (4).

mutants were also found to be sensitive for growth in the presence
of base analogues. A possible explanation for this observation is that
with the loss of strand discrimination endonucleolytic cuts are made
in both parental and daughter strands at mismatch sites. Following
this reasoning Glickman and Radman, (in preparation; Radman et al.,
1978) isolated base analogue resistant revertants of *dam*-strains. This
approach allowed the isolation of hundreds of apparent mutators
which, upon further examination, mapped to the known mutator
sites *mut H, mut S* and *mut L* on the *E. coli* chromosome (Radman
et al., 1978; Glickman and Radman, in preparation).

Further characterization of these mutants supported the original
hypothesis that the base analogue resistant revertants would be
defective in a correndonuclease as the correction of λ-heteroduplex
DNA in these strains is reduced (Rydberg, 1978; Meselson, personal
communication); similar results were found for ∅ M13 heteroduplexes
(Glickman, unpublished observation).

The contribution of mismatch correction in the maintenance of
low error rates during DNA replication is significant. It represents
an increase in accuracy of at least 2 orders of magnitude (see
Table 3). Interestingly, all of the mutators suspected of being
defective in mismatch repair show the same spontaneous mutagenic
spectrum (Cox, 1976; Glickman, 1979) including greatly increased
rates of transitions and, to a lesser extent, an increase in frame shifts.
This latter observation suggests the possibility that the mismatch
correction system may play a role in the correction of frame shifts.
Alternatively, the replication of unrepaired mismatches may lead
to frame shifts.

Table 3. Spontaneous mutation rates of *E. coli* carrying mutations affecting the
correction of mismatched bases. The low error rate of DNA replication in *E. coli*
($\pm 10^{-10}$ errors per nucleotide per replication) is at least partially accounted for
by this post-replicative error-avoidance mechanism which increases the final
fidelity of replication by two to three orders of magnitude. An hypothetical
scheme for post-replicative error-avoidance is presented in Figure 4.

Strain	Relevant genotype	Mutation rates per generation $\times 10^{10}$			
		Str^r	Val^r	Nal^r	Rif^r
KMBL 3752	wild type	0.54	45	3.0	25
KMBL 3754	*dam-4*	8.3	2600	250	930
KMBL 3773	*mutH101*	79	60000	1500	4900
KMBL 3774	*mutL101*	89	21000	1300	49000
KMBL 3775	*mutS101*	4.0	2800	880	2600

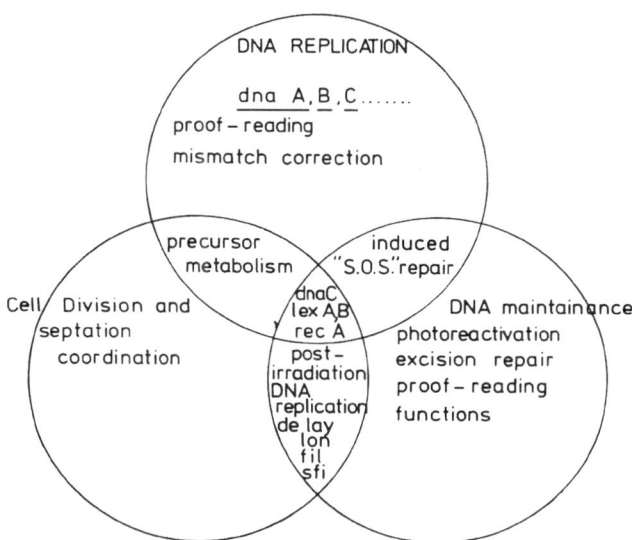

Figure 5. The cellular processes of DNA replication, DNA repair and cell division are intimately inter-related. The complexity of the interdependence of these essential cellular functions is represented by the three overlapping circles.

Evidence from studies involving SV40 DNA (Lai and Nathans, 1975; Wilson, 1977) and polyoma DNA (Miller et al., 1976) suggest the occurrence of mismatch repair in mammalian cells. While newly synthesized DNA is undermethylated (Adams, 1974) the primary methylated base is 5-methylcytosine rather than adenine. The occurrence of mismatch correction, however, is indicative of the existence of some mechanism by which parental and daughter strands can be distinguished.

8. MUTAGENESIS, DNA REPAIR AND CANCER: A SYNTHESIS

DNA replicational fidelity and the ability of cells to survive chemical and physical insult is directly related to a cell's DNA repair capacity. These processes are complex; error-free and error-prone pathways are inter-dependent and are related to other cellular processes such as DNA replication and cell division (Figure 5). In the case of XP, mutagenesis is increased following treatments to which the cells are sensitive. However, AT and FA cells are hypomutable by those agents causing DNA damage which is unrepaired in these cells. One cannot therefore unequivocally state that the induction of mutation is the cause of the increase in cancer observed in FA and AT carriers. Yet we also know that there is a high degree of correlation between mutagenicity and carcinogenicity (McCann et al., 1975; Meselson and Russell, 1977). More fitting, however, with our present information, is that persistent unrepaired DNA lesions can lead either to mutagenesis (error-prone repair at a micro-level) or chromosomal aberrations (tolerance repair at a macro-level) — both of which can potentiate a tumourigenic event.

9. PROMOTION AND THE MUTATIONAL THEORY OF THE ORIGIN OF CANCER

The induction of tumours is a multistep process (for a review see Boutwell, 1974; Miller, 1978) which can be divided into an initiation step involving the irreversible action of a carcinogen and a second stage, promotion, which can occur weeks, months and even years after initiation. The active agent of the classical promoting agent, croton oil, are the 12, 13-diesters of the diterpene alcohol phorbol (Hecker, 1971; Van Duuren, 1976). Recently, Kinsella and Radman (1978) have shown the tumour promoting agent, 12-0-tetrade-canolylphorbol-13-acetate (TPA), to induce sister chromatid exchanges. It is their belief that promoting agents may induce recombinogenic activity. They suggest that mitotic recombination, as well as other "aberrant" mitotic segregations, may account for promotion by the conversion of the initial recessive mutational event in a heterozygous state into a homozygous situation. Moreover, the inducibility of recombination in eukaryotes has been demonstrated in yeast (Fahre and Roman, 1977) and *Ustilago maydis* (Holliday, 1975).

10. CONCLUSIONS

Our still incomplete picture of carcinogenesis is already being applied to the problem of reducing the incidence of cancer. Numerous short-term testing systems have been developed allowing the detection of potential hazards. Problems of how to avoid "false-negative" and "false-positive" results and how to predict with increased probability what agents might be carcinogenic are being intensely studied. Moreover, an improved understanding of the mechanism of tumour promotion may provide a second line of prophylaxis.

Problems of risk extrapolation to man are also receiving serious attention. New inroads are being made into the area of effective dosimetry of chemical carcinogens (Sega et al., 1974; Aaron and Lee, 1978; Aaron et al., 1978; Mohn et al., 1978), which will eventually allow interspecies comparisons on a molecular basis.

ACKNOWLEDGEMENTS

The author wishes to express his appreciation to M. Radman (Brussels), G. Villani (Palo Alto), L. Loeb (Seattle), M.C. Paterson (Chalk River), M.R.M. Schaaper (Leiden) and D. Bootsma (Rotterdam) for their stimulating discussions and, in several cases, for making available preprints of their work. Appreciation is also due to N. Guijt, G. Todd, C. Fijn van Draat and J. Glickman for assistance during the preparation of this manuscript. This work was supported by EURATOM contract BIAN T102-72-1 and the J.A. Cohen Institute for Radiopathology and Radiation Protection.

REFERENCES

Aaron, C.S. and W.R. Lee (1978). Molecular dosimetry of the mutagen ethyl methanosulfonate in *Drosophila melanogaster* spermatozoa: linear relation of DNA alkylation per sperm cell (DOSE) to sex-linked recessive lethals. Mutation Res. 49: 27-44.
Aaron, C.S., A.A. van Zeeland, G.R. Mohn, A.T. Natarajan, A.D. Tates and B.W. Glickman (1978). Quantitative comparative molecular dosimetry of ethyl methanesulfonate in V-79 Chinese hamster cells. *Escherichia coli* and mouse spermatocytes and bone marrow. Abstract VIII Annual Europ. Environ. Mutagen. Society (Dublin). Mutation Res. (in press).
Aaronson, S.A. and Lytle, C.D. (1970). Decreased host cell reactivation of irradiated SV40 virus in xeroderma pigmentosum. Nature 228: 359-361.
Abdulnur, S.F. and R.L. Flurry, Jr. (1976). Effect of guanine alkylation on mispairing Nature 264: 369-370.
Adams, R.L.P. (1974). Newly synthesized DNA is not methylated. Biochim. Biophys. Acta. 335: 365-373.
Arlett, C.F. (1977). Lethal response to DNA damaging agents in a variety of human fibroblast cell strains. Mutation Res. 46: 106.
Auerbach, C. and Robson, J.M. (1947). The production of mutations by chemical substances. Proc. Roy. Soc. Edinburgh B62: 271-283.
Blot, W.J., T.J. Mason, R. Hoover and J.F. Fraumeni Jr. (1977). Cancer by county: Etiologic implications. In "Origins of Human Cancer", Book A, H.H. Hiatt, J.D. Watson, J.A. Winsten, eds., Cold Spring Harbor Laboratories, Cold Spring Harbor, N.Y., pp. 21-32.
Bockstahler, L.E. and C.D. Lytle (1970). Ultraviolet Light Enhanced Reactivation of a Mammalian Virus. Biochem. Biophys. Res. Commun. 41: 184-189.
Bockstahler, L.E. and C.D. Lytle (1971). X-ray enhanced reactivation of ultraviolet irradiated human virus. J. of Virol. 8: 601-602.

Bockstahler, L.E. and C.D. Lytle (1977). Radiation enhanced reactivation of nuclear replicating mammalian viruses. Photochem. Photobiol. 25: 477-482.

Bootsma, D. (1978). Xeroderma pigmentosum. In "DNA repair mechanisms", P.C. Hanawalt, E.C. Friedberg and C.F. Fox, eds., Academic Press, N.Y. (in press).

Boutwell, R.K. (1974). The function and mechanism of promoters of carcinogenesis. CRC. Crit. Rev. Toxiol. 2: 419-443.

Bridges, B.A. (1976). Bacterial Reaction to Radiation, Patterns in Progress. Meadowfield Press Ltd., Durham, England.

Bridges, B.A., R.P. Mottershead and S.G. Sedgwick (1976). Mutagenic DNA repair in Escherichia coli: III. Requirement for a function of DNA polymerase III in ultraviolet-light mutagenesis. Mol. Gen. Genet., 144: 53-58.

Brutlag, D. and A. Kornberg (1972). Enzymatic synthesis of deoxyribonucleic acids. XXXVI. A proofreading function for the 3'-5' exonuclease activity in DNA polymerases. J. Biol. Chem. 247: 241-248.

Cleaver, J.E. (1968). Defective repair replication of DNA in xeroderma pigmentosum. Nature, London. 218: 652-656.

Cleaver, J.E. (1969). Xeroderma pigmentosum: A human disease in which an initial stage of DNA repair is defective. Proc. Nat. Acad. Sci. 63: 428-435.

Cleaver, J.E. (1970). DNA damage and repair in light-sensitive human skin disease. J. Invest. Dermatol. 54: 181-196.

Cleaver, J.E. and J.E. Trosko (1970). Absence of excision of ultraviolet induced cyclobutane dimers in xeroderma pigmentosum. Photochem. Photobiol. 11: 547-550.

Cleaver, J.E. (1972). Xeroderma pigmentosum: Variants with normal DNA repair and normal sensitivity to ultraviolet light. J. Invest. Dermatol. 58: 124-128.

Cleaver, J.E. (1977). DNA repair processes and their impairment in some human diseases. In "Progress in Genetic Toxicology", D. Scott, B.A. Bridges and F.H. Sobels, eds., Elsevier/North Holland, pp. 29-42.

Cleaver, J.E. and D. Bootsma (1975). Xeroderma pigmentosum: Biochemical and genetic characteristics. Ann. Rev. Genet. 9: 19.

Cleaver, J.E. (1978). Xeroderma pigmentosum. In "The metabolic basis of inherited disease", Stanbury, J., J. Wijngaarden and D. Fredrickson, eds., McGraw Hill, New York, pp. 1072-1095.

Cook, K., E.C. Friedberg and J.E. Cleaver (1975). Excision of thymine dimers from specifically incised DNA by extracts of xeroderma pigmentosum cells. Nature 256: 235-236.

Cox, E.C. (1976). Bacterial mutation genes and the control of spontaneous mutation. Ann. Rev. Genet. 10: 135-156.

Craddock, V.M. (1973). The pattern of methylated purines formed in DNA of intact and regenerating liver of rats treated with the carcinogen dimethylnitrosamine. Biochim. Biophys. Acta 312: 202-210.

Cunliffe, P.N., J.R. Mann, A.H. Cameron, K.D. Roberts and H.W.C. Ward (1975). Radiosensitivity in ataxia telangiextasia. Brit. J. Radiol. 48: 374-376.

Day, R.S. III (1974). Studies on repair of adenovirus 2 by human fibroblasts using normal, xeroderma pigmentosum and xeroderma pigmentosum heterozygous strains. Cancer Res. 34: 1965-1970.

Day, R.S. III (1974). Cellular reactivation of ultraviolet irradiated human adenovirus 2 in normal and xeroderma pigmentosum fibroblasts. Photochem. Photobiol. 19: 9-13.

Drake, J.W. and R.H. Baltz (1976). The biochemistry of mutagenesis. Ann. Rev. Biochem. 45: 11-37.

Emmett, E.A. (1973). Ultraviolet light as a cause of skin tumors. CRC Crit. Rev. Toxicol. 2: 211-255.

Fabre, F. and H. Roman (1977). Genetic evidence for inducibility of recombination competence in yeast. Proc. Nat. Acad. Sci. USA 74: 1667-1671.

Finkelberg, R., M. Buchwald and L. Siminovitch (1977). Decreased mutagenesis in cells from Fanconi's anemia patients. Am. J. Human Genetics 29: 42A.

Fowler, R.G., G.E. Degnen and F.C. Cox (1974). Mutational specificity of a conditional *Escherichia coli* mutator, *mutD5*. Mol. Gen. Genet. 133: 179-191.

Friedberg, E.C., J. Duncan and J.E. Cleaver (1974). A thymine dimer excision nuclease in extracts of human cells. Radiat. Res. 59: 98. (abstr.).

Gerchman, L.L. and D.B. Ludlum (1973). The properties of 0^6-methylguanine in templates for RNA polymerase. Biochim. Biophys. Acta 308: 310-316.

German, J. (1972). Genes which increase chromosomal instability in somatic cells and predispose to cancer. Prog. Med. Genet. 8: 61-101.

Gillin, F.D. and N.G. Nosal (1976). Control of mutation frequency by bacteriophage T4 DNA polymerase. II. Accuracy of nucleotide selection by the L88 mutator, CB 120 antimutator and wild type phage T4 DNA polymerases. J. Biol. Chem. 251: 5225-5232.

Glickman, B.W., van der Elsen, P. and M. Radman (1978). Induced mutagenesis in dam-mutants of *Escherichia coli*: a role for 6-methyladenine residues in mutation avoidance. Molec. Gen. Genet. 103: 307-312.

Glickman, B.W. (1979). Spontaneous mutagenesis in *Escherichia coli* strains lacking 6-methyladenine residues in their DNA: An altered mutational spectrum in dam-mutants. Mutat. Res. 61: 157-165.

Goldstein, S. (1971). The role of DNA repair in aging of cultured fibroblasts from xeroderma pigmentosum and normals. Proc. Soc. Exp. Biol. Med. 137: 730-734.

Goth, R. and M.E. Rajewsky (1974). Persistence of 0^6-ethyl guanine in rat-brain DNA: correlation with nervous system specific carcinogenesis by ethyl nitrosourea. Proc. Nat. Acad. Sci. USA 71: 639-643.

Goth, R. and Rajewsky, M.F. (1974). Molecular and cellular mechanisms associated with pulse-carcinogenesis in the rat nervous system by ethyl-nitrosourea: Ethylation of nucleic acids and elimination rates of ethylated bases from the DNA of different tissues. Z. Krebsforsch., 82: 37-64.

Grossman, L., A. Braun, R. Feldberg and I. Mahler (1975). Enzymatic repair of DNA. Ann. Rev. Biochemistry 44: 19-43.

Haenszel, W. and Kurihara, M. (1968). Studies of Japanese migrates. I. Mortality from cancer and other diseases among Japanese in the United States. J. Nat. Cancer Inst. 40: 43-68.

Haenszel, W., J.W. Berg, M. Segi, M. Kurihara and F. Locke (1973). Large bowel cancer in Hawaiian Japanese. J. Nat. Cancer Inst. 51: 1765-1779.

Haenszel, W. (1975). Migrant Studies. In "Persons at High Risk of Cancer. An Approach to Cancer Etiology and Control", J.F. Fraumeni Jr., ed., Academic Press, Inc., New York, pp. 361-371.

Hart, R.W. and R.B. Setlow (1975). Direct evidence that pyrimidine dimers in DNA in neoplastic transformation. In "Molecular mechanisms for repair of DNA", part B, P.C. Hanawalt and R.B. Setlow, eds. Plenum Press, New York, pp. 719-724.

Haynes, R.H. (1966). General discussion. Radiat. Res. (Suppl. 6). 232.

Hecker, E. (1971). Isolation and characterization of the cocarcinogenic principles from croton oil. Methods Cancer Res. 6: 439-484.

Higginson, J. (1969). Present trends in cancer epidemiology. Can. Cancer Conf. 8: 40-75.

Higurashi, M. and P.E. Coenen (1973). In vitro chromosomal radiosensitivity in "chromosomal breakage syndromes". Cancer 32: 380-383.

Hoar, D.I. and P. Sargeant (1976). Chemical Mutagen Hypersensitivity in Ataxia

Telangiectasia. Nature 261: 590-592.
Holliday, R. (1975). Further evidence for an inducible recombination repair system in *Ustilago maydis*. Mutation Res. 29: 149-153.
Ishii, Y. and S. Kondo (1975). Comparative analysis of deletion and base charge mutabilities of *Escherichia coli* B strains differing in DNA repair capacity (wild type, uvra-, pola-, reca-) by various mutagens. Mutation Res. 27: 27-44.
Jahn, E.L. and G.W. Litman (1977). Distribution of Covalently Bound Benzo(a) pyrene in Chromatin. Biochim. Biophys. Res. Commun. 76: 534-540.
Kato, H. and H.F. Stich (1976). Sister chromatid exchanges in ageing and repair-deficient human fibroblasts. Nature 260: 447-448.
Kimball, R.F. (1978). The relation of repair phenomena to mutation induction in bacteria. Mutation Res. (in press).
Kinsella, A. and Radman, M. (1978). Tumor promoter induces sister chromatid exchanges: relevance to mechanisms of carcinogenesis. Proc. Nat. Acad. Sci. USA (in press).
Kirtikar, D.M. and D.A. Goldthwait (1974). The enzymatic release of 0^6-methyl-guanine and 3-methyladenine from DNA reacted with the carcinogen N-methyl-N-nitrosourea. Proc. Nat. Acad. Sci. USA 71: 2022-2026.
Kleihaus, R. and P.N. Magee (1973). Alkylation of rat brain nucleic acids by N-methyl-N-nitrosourea and methylmethanesulfonate. J. Neurochem. 20: 595-600.
Kleihaus, P. and G.P. Margison (1974). Carcinogenicity of N-methyl-N-nitrosourea: possible role of repair excision of 0^6-methylguanine from DNA. J. Nat. Cancer Inst. 53: 1839-1841.
Kleihaus, P. and G.P. Margison (1976). Exhaustion and recovery of repair excision of 0^6-methyl guanine from rat liver DNA. Nature 259: 153-155.
Kornberg, R.D. (1977). Structure of chromatin. Ann. Rev. Biochem. 46: 931-954.
Kraemer, K.H., E.A. de Weerd-Kastelein, J.H. Robbins, W. Keijzer, S.F. Barrett, R.A. Petinga and D. Bootsma (1975). Five complementation groups in xeroderma pigmentosum. Mutation Res. 33: 327-340.
Kraemer, K.H., H.G. Coon, R.A. Petinga, S.F. Barrett, A.E. Rahe and J.H. Robbins (1975). Genetic heterogenicity in xeroderma pigmentosum: complementation groups and their relationship to DNA repair rates. Proc. Nat. Acad. Sci. 72: 59-63.
Kraemer, K.H. (1977). Ataxia telangiectasia. In "Cellular Senescence and Somatic Cell Genetics: DNA Repair Processes", W.W. Nichols and D.G. Murphy, eds., Symposia Specialists, Miami, pp. 37-71.
Kuhnlein, U., E.E. Penhoet and S. Linn (1976). An altered apurinic DNA endonu-clease activity in group A and group D xeroderma pigmentosum fibroblasts. Proc. Nat. Acad. Sci. USA 73: 1169-1173.
Kuhnlein, U., B. Lee, E.E. Penhoet and S. Linn (1978). Xeroderma pigmentosum fibroblasts of the D group lack an apurinic DNA endonuclease species with a low apprent K_m. Nuc. Acids. Res. 5: 951-960.
Lacks, S. and B. Greenberg (1977). Complementary specificity of restriction endonucleases of *Diplococcus pneumoniae* with respect to DNA methylation. J. Molec. Biol. 114: 153-168.
Lai, C. and D. Nathans (1975). A map of temperature-sensitive mutants of simian virus 40. Virology 66: 70-81.
Latt, S.A., G. Stetten, L.A. Juergens, G.R. Buchanan and P.S. Gerald (1975). Induction by Alkylating Agents of Sister Chromatid Exchanges and Chromatid Breaks in Fanconi's Anemia. Proc. Nat. Acad. Sci. USA 72: 4066-4070.
Lavin, M.F., P.C. Chen and C. Kidsen (1978). Ataxia Telangiectasia: Characterization of Heterozygotes. J. Supramol. Struct., suppl. 2: 75-75.

Lawley, P.D. and C.J. Thatcher (1970). Methylation of deoxyribonucleic acid in cultured mammalian cells by N-methyl-N'-nitro-nitrosoguanidine. Biochem. J. 116: 693-707.

Lawley, P.D. and S.A. Shah (1972). Methylation of ribonucleic acid by the carcinogenes dimethylsulfate, N-methyl-N-nitrosourea and N-methyl-N'-nitro-N-nitrosoguanidine. Biochem. J. 128: 177-132.

Lawley, P.D., D.J. Orr, S.A. Shah, P.B. Farmer and M. Jarman (1972). Reaction products from N-methyl-N-nitrosourea and deoxyribonucleic acid containing thymidine residues synthesis and identification of a new methylation product, 0^4-methyl thymidine. Biochem. J. 135: 193-201.

Lehmann, A.R. (1972). Post replication repair of DNA in ultraviolet irradiated mammalian cells. J. Mol. Biol. 66: 319-337.

Lehmann, A.R. S. Kirk-Bell, C.F. Arlett, M.C. Paterson, P.H.M. Lohman, E.A. de Weerd-Kastelein and D. Bootsma (1975). Xeroderma pigmentosum cells with normal levels of excision repair have a defect in DNA synthesis after UV-irradiation. Proc. Nat. Acad. Sci. 72: 219-223.

Lehmann, A.R. and B.A. Bridges (1977). DNA repair. In "Essays in Biochemistry", P.N. Campbell and W.N. Aldridge, eds., Academic Press, pp. 71-119.

Lehmann, A.R. and Stevens, S. (1977). The production and repair of double strand breaks in cells from normal humans and from patients with ataxia telangiectasia. Biochim. Biophys. Acta 474: 49-60.

Ludlum, D.B. (1970). The properties of 7-methylguanine-containing templates for ribonucleic acid polymerase. J. Biol. Chem. 245: 477-482.

Lytle, C.D., S.A. Aaronson and E. Harvy (1972). Host cell reactivation in mammalian cells. II. Survival of herpes simplex virus and vaccinia virus in normal human and xeroderma pigmentosum cells. Int. J. Radiat. Biol. 22: 159-165.

Maher, V.M. and J.J. McCormick (1975). Effect of DNA repair on the cytotoxicity and on the frequency of mutations induced in normal human skin fibroblasts and in strains of xeroderma pigmentosum by ultraviolet irradiation and by chemical carcinogens. In "International Symposium Protein and Other Adducts to DNA: Their significance to aging, carcinogenesis and radiation biology", Energy Research and Development Administration. National Cancer Institute and National Science Foundation Washington D.C. (abstr.), p. 83.

Maher, V.M., L.M Ouellette, R.D. Curren and J.J. McCormick (1976). Frequency of ultraviolet light induced mutation is higher in xeroderma pigmentosum variant cells. Nature 261: 593-595.

Marinus, M.G. and R.N. Morris (1974). Biological function for the 6-methyladenine residues in the DNA of Escherichia coli K12. J. Molec. Biol. 85: 309-322.

Marinus, M.G. and N.R. Morris (1975). Pleiotropic effects of a DNA adenine methylation mutation (dam-3) in Escherichia coli K12. Mutation Res. 28: 15-26.

McCann, J., E. Choi, E. Yamasaki and B.N. Ames (1975). Detection of carcinogens as mutagens in the Salmonella/microsome test: Assay of 300 chemicals. Proc. Nat. Acad. Sci. USA 72: 5135-5139.

McCann, J., N.N. Spingarn, J. Kobori and B.N. Ames (1975). Detection of carcinogens as mutagens: bacterial tester strains with R factor plasmids. Proc. Nat. Acid. Sci. USA 72: 979-983.

Meselsen, M. and K. Russell (1977). Comparisons of carcinogenic and mutagenic potency. In "Origins of Human Cancers", Book C. H.H. Hiatt, J.D. Watson and J.A. Winsten, eds., Cold Spring Harbor Laboratory, Cold Spring Harbor, New York, pp. 1473-1481.

Metzger, G., F.X. Wilhelm and M.L. Wilhelm (1977). Non-random Binding of a Chemical Carcinogen to the DNA in Chromatin. Biophys. Biochem. Res. Commun. 75: 703-710.

Miller, E.C. (1978). Some current perspectives on chemical carcinogenesis in humans and experimental animals: Presidential address. Cancer Research 38: 1479-1496.

Miller, L.K., B.E. Cooke and H. Fried (1976). Fate of mismatched base-pair regions in polyoma heteroduplex DNA during infection of mouse cells. Proc. Nat. Acad. Sci. USA 73: 3073-3077.

Mortelman, K., E.C. Friedberg, H. Slcr, G. Thomas and J.E. Cleaver (1976). Defective thymine dimer excision by cell-free extracts of xeroderma pigmentosum cells. Proc. Nat. Acad. Sci. 73: 2757-2761.

Mohn, G.R., A.A. van Zeeland, B.W. Glickman, A.T. Natarajan and C.S. Aaron (1978). Quantitative molecular dosimetry of ethyl methanosulphonate (EMS) in several genetic test systems. In "Short term mutagenicity test systems for the detection of carcinogens", Dortmund, 15-17 November.

Moses, H.L., R.A. Wekster, G.D. Martin and T.C. Spelsberg (1976). Binding of Polycyclic Aromatic Hydrocarbons to Transcriptionally Active Nuclear Subfractions of AKR Mouse Embryo Cells. Cancer Res. 36: 2905-2910.

Mount, D.W. (1977). A mutant of E. coli showing constitutive expression of the lysogenic induction and error-prone DNA repair pathways. Proc. Nat. Acad. Sci. USA 74: 300-304.

Nicoll, J.W., P.F. Swann and A.E. Pegg (1975). Effect of dimethyl nitrosamine on persistence of methylated guanines in rat liver and kidney DNA. Nature 254: 261-262.

Oudet, P., M. Gross-Bellard and P. Chambon (1975). Electron microscope and biochemical evidence that chromatin structure is a repeating unit. Cell 4: 281-300.

Oishi, M., C.L. Smith and B. Friefeld (1972). The molecular events and molecules which lead to induction of prophage and SOS function. CSHS QS 43 (in press).

Painter, R.B. and B.R. Young (1972). Repair replication in mammalian cells after X-irradiation. Mutat. Res. 14: 225-235.

Paterson, M.C., P.H.M. Lohman and M.L. Sluyter (1973). Use of a UV-endonuclease from Micrococcus luteus to monitor the progress of DNA repair in UV-irradiated human cells. Mutat. Res. 19: 245-256.

Paterson, M.C., B.P. Smith, P.H.M. Lohman, A.K. Anderson and L. Fishman (1976). Defective excision repair of γ-ray damaged DNA in human (ataxia telangiectasia) fibroblasts. Nature 260: 444-446.

Paterson, M.C. (1978). Environmental carcinogenesis and imperfect repair of damaged DNA in Homo sapiens causal relation revealed by rare hereditary disorder. In "Carcinogens: identification and mechanisms of action", Thirty-first Annual Symposium on Fundamental Cancer Research, The University of Texas System Cancer Center, Houston, Texas, 1978 on March 1-3, C.R. Shaw and A.C. Griffin, eds., Academic Press, New York.

Paterson, M.C., B.P. Smith, P.J. Smith and A.K. Anderson (1978). Abstract. Radiat. Res. 74: 83-84.

Poon, P.K., R.L. O'Brien and J.W. Parker (1974). Defective DNA repair in Fanconi's anaemia. Nature 250: 223-225.

Rabson, A.S., S.A. Tyrrell and F.Y. Legallais (1969). Growth of ultraviolet damaged herpes virus in xeroderma pigmentosum cells. Proc. Soc. Exp. Biol. Med. 132: 802-806.

Radman, M. (1975). SOS repair hypothesis: phenomenology of inducible repair which is accompanied by mutagenesis. In "Molecular mechanism for the repair of DNA", P.C. Hanawalt, R.B. Setlow, eds., Plenum Press, New York, pp. 355-367.

Radman, M., G. Villani, S. Boiteux, M. Defais, P. Caillet-Fauquet and S. Spidari

(1977). On the molecular mechanism of induced mutagenesis. In "Origins of human cancer", H. Hiatt, J.D. Watson, and J.D. Winstein, eds., Cold Spring Harbor Laboratory, Cold Spring Harbor, New York.

Radman, M., S. Spadari and G. Villani (1978). Ultraviolet induced mutagenesis and carcinogenesis: many hypotheses for few results. J. Natl. Cancer Inst. Monogr. 50 (in press).

Radman, M., G. Villani, S. Boiteux, A.R. Kinsella, B.W. Glickman and S. Spadari (1978). Replicational fidelity: mechanisms of mutation avoidance and mutation fixation. Cold Harbor Symposium in Quant. Biol. 43 (in press).

Rajewsky, M.F., R. Goth, O.D. Laerum, H. Biessmann and D.F. Hülser (1976). Molecular and cellular mechanisms in nervous system-specific carcinogenesis by N-ethyl-N-nitrosourea. In "Fundamentals in cancer prevention", P.N. Magee et al., eds., University of Tokyo Press/University Park Press, Baltimore, Maryland, p. 313.

Ramanathon, R., S. Rajalakshmi, D.S.R. Sarma and E. Farber (1976). Nonrandom nature of in vivo methylation by dimethylnitrosamine and the subsequent removal of methylated products from rat liver chromatin DNA. Cancer Res. 36: 2073-2079.

Regan, J.D. and R.B. Setlow (1974). Two forms of repair in the DNA of human cells, damaged by chemical carcinogens and mutagens. Cancer Res. 34: 3318-3325.

Robbins, J.H., K.H. Kraemer, M.A. Lutzner, B.W. Festoff and H.G. Coon (1974). Xeroderma pigmentosum. An inherited disease with sun sensitivity, multiple cutaneous neoplasma and abnormal DNA repair. Ann. Int. Med. 80: 221-248.

Roberts, J.W., C.W. Roberts and D.W. Mount (1977). Proteolytic Cleavage of Bacteriophage Lambda Repressor in Induction. Proc. Nat. Acad. Sci. 72: 147-151.

Roberts, J.W., C.W. Roberts and N.L. Craig (1978). The E. coli RecA gene product inactivates phage lambda repressor. CSHSQB, 43 (in press).

Rydberg, B. (1978). Bromouracil mutagenesis and mismatch repair in mutator strains of Escherichia coli. Mutation Res. 52: 11-24.

Rykowski, M., P. Pukkila, M. Radman, R. Wagner and M.S. Meselson (1978). Undermethylation and strand selection in DNA mismatch repair (Abstract Book). Cold Spring Harbour Symposium on Quantitative Biology 43: 128.

Sarasin, A.R. and P.C. Hanawalt (1978). Carcinogens enhance survival of UV-irradiated SV40 in treated monkey kidney cells; Induction of a recovery pathway? Proc. Natl. Acad. Sci. USA 75: 346-350.

Sasaki, M.S. and A. Tonomura (1973). A high susceptibility of Fanconi's anaemia to chromosome breakage by DNA cross-linking agents. Cancer Res. 33: 1829-1836.

Scudiero, D.A. (1978). Repair Deficiency in N-Methyl-N'-Nitro-N-Nitrosoguanide Treated Ataxia Telangiectasia (AT) Fibroblasts. J. Supramol. Struct., suppl. 2: 83-83.

Sedgwick, R.P. and E. Boder (1972). Ataxia telangiectasia. In "Handbook of Clinical Neurology", P.J. Vinken and G.W. Bruyn, eds., Vol. 14, North Holland Publ. Co., Amsterdam, pp. 267-339.

Sega, G.A., R.B. Cummings and M.F. Walton (1974). Dosimetry studies on the ethylation of mouse sperm DNA after in vivo exposure to ^{3}H ethyl methanesulfonate. Mutation Res. 24: 317-333.

Setlow, R.B., J.D. Regan, J. German and W.L. Carrier (1969). Evidence that xeroderma pigmentosum cells do not perform the first step in the repair of ultraviolet damage to their DNA. Proc. Nat. Acad. Sci. 64: 1035-1041.

Setlow, R.B. (1978). Repair deficient human disorders and cancer. Nature 271: 713-717.

Singer, B. (1975). The chemical effects of nucleic acid alkylation and their relation to mutagenesis and carcinogenesis. Progr. Nucleic Acid Res. Mol. Biol. 15: 219-284.

Singer, B. and H. Fraenkel-Conrat (1975). The specificity of different classes of ethylating agents toward various sites in RNA Biochemistry 14: 722-782.

Singer, B. (1976). All oxygens in nucleic acids react with carcinogenic ethylating agents. Nature, 264: 333-339.

Stich, H.F., R.H.C. San and Y. Kawazone (1973). Increased sensitivity of xeroderma pigmentosum cells to some chemical carcinogens and mutagens. Mutat. Res. 17: 127-137.

Sun, L. and B. Singer (1975). The specificity of different classes of ethylating agents toward various sites of Hela cell DNA in vitro and in vivo. Biochemistry 14: 1795-1802.

Sutherland, B.M. (1974). Photoreactivating enzyme from human leukocytes. Nature 248: 109-112.

Sutherland, B.M., M. Rice and E. Wagner (1975). Xeroderma pigmentosum cells contain low levels of photoreactivating enzyme. Proc. Natl. Acad. Sci. 72: 103-107.

Swift, M. (1971). Fanconi's anaemia in the genetics of neoplasia. Nature 230: 370-373.

Swift, M., L. Sholman, M. Perry and C. Chase (1976). Malignant neoplasms in the families of patients with ataxia telangiectasia. Cancer Res. 36: 209-215.

Takebe, H., J.I. Furuyama, Y. Miki and S. Kondo (1972). High sensitivity of xeroderma pigmentosum cells to the carcinogen 4-nitroquinoline-1-oxide. Mutat. Res. 15: 98-100.

Takebe, H. (1978). Relationship Between DNA Repair Defect and Skin Cancers in Xeroderma Pigmentosum. J. Supramol. Structure, suppl. 2: 30-30.

Tanaka, K., Sekiguchi, M. and Y. Okada. (1975). Restoration of ultraviolet induced unscheduled DNA synthesis of xeroderma pigmentosum cells by the concomitant treatment with bacteriophage T4 endonuclease V and HVJ (Sendai virus). Proc. Nat. Acad. Sci. USA 72: 4071-4075.

Taylor, A.M.R., D.G. Harnden, C.F. Arlett, S.A. Harcourt, A.R. Lehmann, S. Stevens and B.A. Bridges (1975). Ataxia telangiectasia: a human mutation with abnormal radiation sensitivity. Nature 258: 427-429.

Taylor, A.M.R., J.A. Metcalfe, J.M. Oxford and D.G. Harnden (1976). Is chromatid-type damage in ataxia telangiectasia after irradiation at G_0 a consequence of defective repair? Nature 260: 441-443.

Topal, M.D. and J.R. Fresco (1976). Complementary base pairing and the origin of substitution mutations. Nature 263: 285-293.

Urbach, F., D.B. Rose and M. Bonnem (1972). Genetic and environmental interactions in skin carcinogenesis. In "Environment and Cancer", M.D. Anderson Hospital and Tumor Institute, Williams and Witkins, Baltimore, pp. 354-371.

Van Duren, B.L. (1976). Tumor-promoting and co-carcinogenic agents in chemical carcinogenesis. In "Chemical Carcinogens", American Chemical Society Monograph no. 73, C.E. Searle, ed., American Chemical Society, Washington, D.C., pp. 24-51.

Villani, G. (1978). Les rôles des DNA polymerases dans la mutagenèse induite. Ph.D. Thesis. University of Brussels.

Villani, G., S. Boiteux and M. Radman (1978). Mechanisms of ultraviolet-induced mutagenesis extent and fidelity of in vitro DNA-synthesis on irradiated templates. Proc. Natl. Acad. Sci. USA 75: 3037-3041.

Wager, R. Jr. and M. Meselson (1976). Repair tracts in mismatched DNA heteroduplexes. Proc. Nat. Acad. Sci (Wash.) 73: 4135-4139.

Walker, J.G. and D.F. Ewart (1973). The nature of single-strand breaks in DNA following treatment of L-cells with methylating agents. Mutation Res. 19: 331-341.

Watson, J.D., F.H.C. Crick (1953). A structure for deoxyribose nucleic acids. Nature 171: 737-738.

Weisbach, A. Eukaryotic DNA polymerases. Ann. Rev. Biochem. 46: 25-47.

Wilson, J.H. (1977). Genetic analysis of host range mutant viruses suggests an uncoating defect in simian virus 40-resistant monkey cells. Proc. Nat. Acad. Sci. (Washington) 74: 3503-3507.

Witkin, E.M. (1974). Thermal enhancement of ultraviolet mobility in a *tif-1 uvrA* derivative of *Escherichia coli* B/r: evidence that ultraviolet mutagenesis depends upon an inducible function. Proc. Nat. Acad. Sci. 71: 1930-1934.

Witkin, E.M. (1976). Ultraviolet mutagenesis and inducible DNA repair in *Escherichia coli*. Bact. Rev. 40: 869-907.

Yarosh, D.B. (1978). Enzymatic pathway of error-prone repair in UV-irradiated phage T4. J. Supramol. Struct., suppl. 2, p. 69.

Závadová. A. (1971). Host cell repair of vaccinia virus and of double stranded RNA of encephalomyocarditis virus. Nature New Biol. 233: 123.

4. RNA TUMOUR VIRUSES: INTERESTING INTERACTIONS WITH THE HOST GENOME

P. BENTVELZEN

ABSTRACT

Horizontally transmitted RNA tumour viruses establish after infection a somatic DNA provirus into cellular DNA. Transcription of the provirus which is under host control usually leads to the synthesis of a 35S RNA molecule, which may: (a) be incorporated in a dimeric form into new virions; (b) serve as messenger for the precursor proteins of the viral core polypeptides and occasionally also for the RNA-dependent DNA polymerase; or (c) be processed into smaller sized messengers for the precursor protein of the viral envelope glycoprotein and of the gene, associated with oncogenic transformation, whose product in a few systems has been described. Host genes may interfere with these processes, often leading to the arrest of neoplastic conversion.

RNA tumour viruses may also be transmitted as genetic factors of the host. Expression of germinal proviruses can be regulated at either the transcriptional or translational level. Mutations in controlling genes or treatment with carcinogens may lead to the release of virus. Highly oncogenic viruses may result of the recombination between different types of such genetically transmitted endogenous viruses.

1. INTRODUCTION

Several spontaneously occurring neoplasms in a great variety of vertebrates are caused by an RNA tumour virus (Gross, 1970; Tooze, 1973). Viruses have also been isolated from human haematological neoplasms which are closely related to viruses that are oncogenic to subhuman primates (Gallagher and Gallo, 1975; Nooter et al., 1975; 1977). These human-derived isolates are oncogenic to animals (Bergholtz et al., 1976; Nooter et al., 1978), supporting the concept of an etiological role of these viruses in human malignancy. With regard to human breast cancer, many suggestions have been made about an

association between this disease and a factor related to the mouse
mammary tumour virus (Axel et al., 1972; Black et al., 1975; Müller
et al., 1976; Cunningham-Rundles et al., 1976; Mesa-Tejada et al.,
1978). On the basis of these studies and recent results obtained in my
own laboratory, I am convinced that a high percentage of human breast
cancers are indeed caused by a virus in interaction with hormonal
and nutritional factors, although mammary carcinoma is not an
infectious disease.

The RNA tumour viruses are important from a veterinarian point of
view (chicken and cattle leukosis), but are also increasingly interesting
in a medical sense as indicated above. These viruses display a number
of highly interesting interactions with the host genome, that even
when they were clinically irrelevant, they would be valuable tools for
the study of several biological processes in eukaryotic systems.

2. STRUCTURE OF RNA TUMOUR VIRUSES

The RNA tumour viruses belong to the group of Retroviridae (Fenner,
1976), which are characterized by containing the enzyme RNA-
dependent DNA-polymerase, better known as reverse transcriptase. So
far, they comprise two genera of this family: Oncovirus B and C. The
separation between both genera has been originally made on morphological grounds (Bernhard, 1958). The prototype of oncovirus B is the
murine mammary tumour virus (Figure 1). Several other viral isolates
from a variety of animal species have been wrongly classified under
this genus (Schildlovsky, 1977). Unfortunately, as yet no decent
electronmicroscopic picture has been presented of a presumed B-
type oncovirus detected in human material.

Viruses belonging to the genus oncovirus C (Figure 1) are predominantly involved in the genesis of sarcomas, lymphomas or leukemias,
although some avian viruses might also cause carcinomas (Langlois
et al., 1970). C-type oncoviruses have been isolated from chickens,
mice, cats, hamsters, monkeys and human beings. Viruses with the
same morphology have also been isolated from tissues of many other
vertebrates, but their oncogenic potential remains to be established.

The most striking morphological difference between true B-type
and C-type oncoviruses is the smaller size and excentric location of the
electron-dense nucleoid (core) in the first group. The B-type viruses
contain also more prominent protrusions (spikes) of the viral envelope,
which is constituted of glycoproteins and phospholipids.

The polypeptides of most known RNA tumour viruses have been

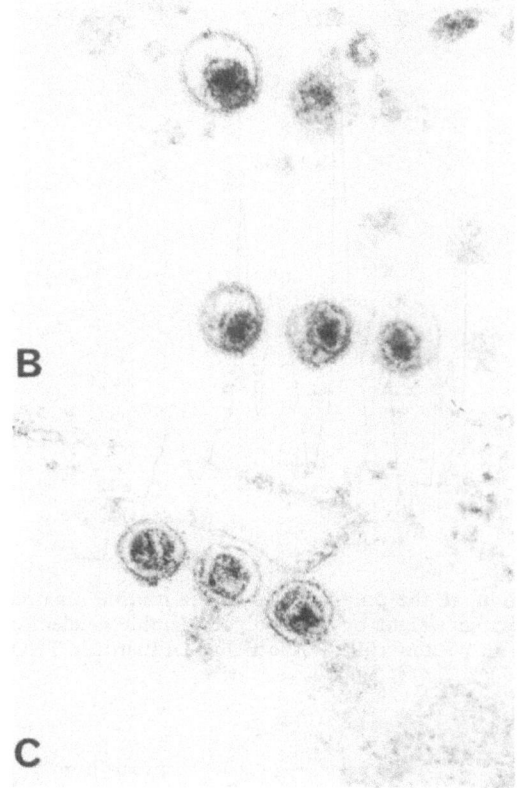

Figure 1. Electron micrographs of RNA tumour viruses (100 x). Upper: B-type oncovirus, the murine mammary tumour virus. Lower: C-type oncovirus, Rauscher murine leukaemia virus. (Photographs taken by F.G. de Groot, Institute for Experimental Gerontology TNO, Rijswijk, The Netherlands).

well characterized. The proteins of the mouse mammary tumour virus (MuMTV) have been separated according to their molecular weight by SDS-poly-acrylamide gelelectrophoresis (Figure 2). The different polypeptides are indicated accordingly; for instance, a protein with a molecular weight of 28,000 is designated as p28 and a glycoprotein with a molecular weight of 52,000 as gp52. The location of the different polypeptides within the virion, as concluded from studies by Cardiff et al. (1974) and results obtained in our own laboratory, is given in Figure 3. A similar scheme has been devised for the C-type oncoviruses (Bolognesi et al., 1978).

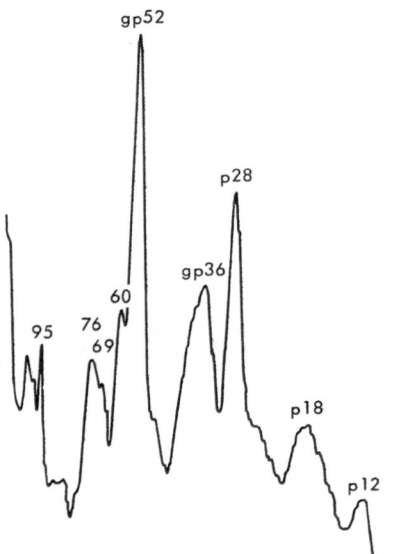

Figure 2. Separation of the polypeptides of the murine mammary tumour virus according to molecular weight by SDS-polyacrylamide gelelectrophoresis (photograph provided by F. Westenbrink, Radiobiological Institute TNO).

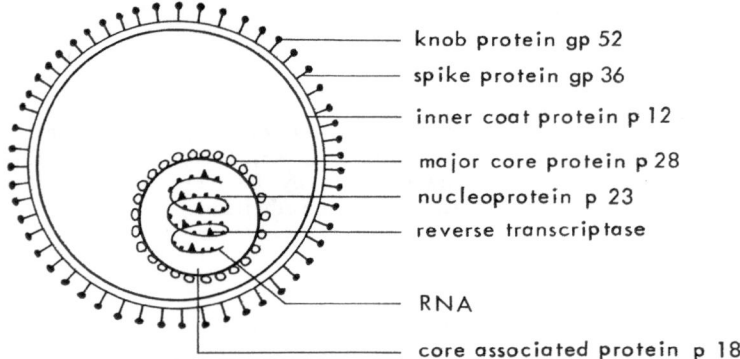

Figure 3. Presumed location of the polypeptides of the murine mammary tumour virus within the virion.

3. GENETIC MAP OF RNA TUMOUR VIRUSES

The genome of retroviruses is a single-stranded RNA molecule, which sediments in sucrose gradients at 60-70S. The genome consists of two identical subunits (Duesberg et al., 1975; Weismann et al., 1975), which are joined together at their 5'-end (Kung et al., 1976).

On the basis of studies in several laboratories with temperature-sensitive or deletion mutants, Baltimore (1975) constructed the following genetic map of oncoviruses.

5'-gag-pol-env-onc-poly Adenine-3'

The *gag*-gene codes for the so-called group-specific antigens, which would be mainly located in the core. This is a somewhat unfortunate nomenclature, since most of these internal polypeptides also carry type-specific antigenic determinants while the polypeptides coded for by the other viral genes also carry some group-specific determinants.

The *pol*-gene codes for the enzyme reverse transcriptase, which can synthesize a DNA copy of an RNA template (Temin and Mizutani, 1970; Baltimore, 1970).

The *env*-gene codes for viral envelope proteins, which usually are glycosylated. In case of MuMTV, a small molecular weight polypeptide in the viral membrane (p12) seems to be coded for by the *gag*-gene (Nusse, personal communication).

The *onc*-gene controls the neoplastic transformation of a cell. The product of this gene of the avian sarcomavirus (ASV) indicated as *src* has recently been analyzed: it is a protein with a molecular weight of 60,000 daltons (Brugge and Erikson, 1977). When cells transformed by a virus with a temperature-sensitive mutation in the *src* gene are kept at a nonpermissive temperature, resulting in a "normal" phenotype of the cells, this protein is lacking. This protein proves to be a protein kinase (Collett and Erikson, 1978). It remains unclear how extensive phosphorylation of proteins would lead to neoplastic conversion.

The *src*-gene product of ASV has so far been characterized as a cytoplasmic protein. In various oncovirus systems evidence has been obtained for the presence on the cell surface of a new antigen which is not present in virus particles but seems to be virally coded (Stephenson et al., 1977; Fenyö et al., 1977; Bentvelzen and Creemers, 1977; Kurth and Kitchener, 1978).

It is very well possible that the *onc*-gene of the different oncoviruses code not only for a cytoplasmic protein kinase but also for a tumour-specific surface antigen. The latter need not have the same molecular weight, but must be antigenically related to the cytoplasmic protein. It is not to be expected that the *onc*-genes of the various RNA tumour viruses would be homologous.

4. LIFE CYCLE OF ONCOVIRUSES

In order to penetrate a cell an interaction of the viral envelope with a specific receptor on the cell surface is needed. When susceptible cells are first incubated with the isolated major viral glycoprotein, subsequent infection with the live virus fails to take place. After penetration, virus uncoating takes place rapidly; a process of which many details remain to be elucidated. Within a few hours the enzyme reverse transcriptase has made a DNA copy of the viral genome. The same enzyme digests the RNA strand, and a DNA copy is produced of the newly formed viral DNA. The DNA moves to the nucleus, becomes circularized and then integrates at a chromosomal site (for a review, see Wu, 1977).

In the MuMTV-system it has been found that the provirus can integrate at various sites, and that the site of integration seems to be irrelevant for neoplastic conversion of a mammary cell (Cohen et al., 1978).

In contrast to the DNA tumour viruses, limitation in virus expression is not needed for the maintenance of the transformed state. In most cell systems RNA tumour viruses are not cytocidal (for the few exceptions, see Bentvelzen, 1974a). On the other hand full expression of the virus is not a prerequisite for neoplastic conversion. Defective strains have been described for several oncoviruses (Hanafusa et al., 1963; Hartly and Rowe, 1966; Graf, 1973; Aaronson, 1973). They, for instance, lack the env-gene. Such virus strains can maintain the neoplastic state of a cell without any synthesis of the env-gene products. Competent ASV can transform mammalian cells without production of complete virus particles (Svoboda and Hlozanek, 1970). The nature of this inhibition in virus replication remains to be established.

Sarcomatogenic viruses can transform a great variety of cell types (Nooter and Bentvelzen, 1977), but the epigenetic state of the cell strongly influences the oncogenic activity of other oncoviruses. The mouse mammary tumour virus can replicate in various organs like salivary gland or prostate, but only transforms mammary cells (Bentvelzen and Brinkhof, 1977). In vitro murine leukaemogenic viruses (MuLV) can replicate in fibroblasts and epithelial cell lines without any sign of transformation, while in vivo these viruses rapidly induce haematological malignancies. Brommer and Bentvelzen (1974) demonstrated a highly subtle interplay between haematological differentiation and the Rauscher leukaemia virus in the induction of erythroleukaemia in mice.

Transcription of the provirus leads usually to the synthesis of 35S RNA, corresponding with a single genomic subunit. This high-molecular weight RNA may become incorporated in a dimeric form in the virion. It may also serve as a messenger for the *gag*-precursor protein, which in several steps is proteolytically cleaved into the structural proteins of the viral core (Van Zaane et al., 1975; Naso et al., 1975). Occasionally a very large read-through protein is made with a molecular weight of approx. 200,000 daltons, which not only contains the *gag*-precursor protein but also the *pol*-gene product (Oppermann et al., 1977; Kopchick et al., 1978). The *gag*-gene products accumulate in the cytoplasm of the cell. Only small amounts are deposited at the cell surface; in that case the products are glycosylated, as has been found for MuLV (Snyder et al., 1977).

The *env*-gene products are synthesized on membrane-bound polysomes, with a messenger considerably smaller than the 35S subunit (Gielkens et al., 1976; Karshin et al., 1977). The *env*-messenger probably results from the enzymatic breakdown of the 35S transcript. The *env*-gene products are present in the cytoplasm in considerably smaller amounts than the viral core polypeptides, but are mainly deposited at the cell surface (Westenbrink et al., 1979). The 35S RNA will be complexed with *gag*-proteins in the cytoplasm. In case of MuMTV, conspicuous morphological structures called A-type particles (Bernhard, 1958) are formed. The complex of viral RNA and proteins moves to sites, containing deposits of viral glycoproteins. Virus particles then bud at such sites from the cell. The newly released virions look like a collection of concentric rings. The virions mature by the formation of an electron-dense core. This process coincides with the proteolytic cleavage of the various precursor proteins (Stephenson et al., 1975; Yeger et al., 1976; Witte and Baltimore, 1978).

It remains to be established whether a separate messenger exists for the gene-product(s) of the various *onc*-genes. If so, the interplay between cell differentiation and oncogenic action of RNA tumour viruses other than the sarcomaviruses could be better understood.

Our present insight into the life cycle of an infectious RNA tumour virus is presented in Figure 4.

5. HOST GENETIC FACTORS INTERFERING WITH THE ONCOGENIC ACTION OF EXOGENOUS VIRUSES

The aforementioned life cycle holds for ordinary infectious viruses. It

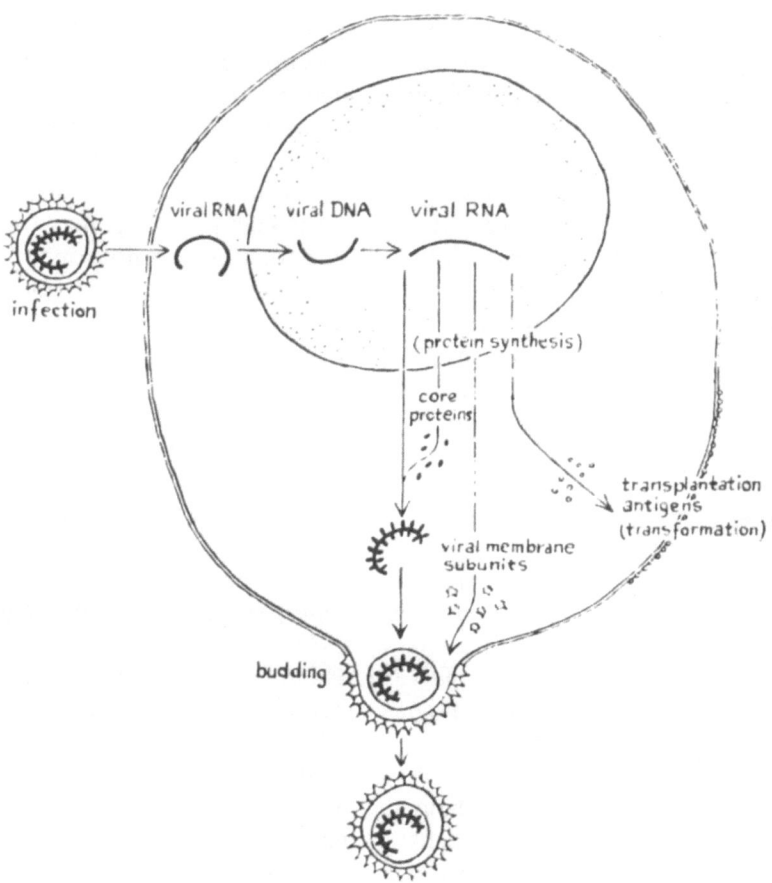

Figure 4. Life-cycle of an infectious RNA tumour virus.

seems that several haematological neoplasms in chickens, cats and
cattle are caused by such horizontally transmitted viruses. Childhood
leukaemia in man also seems to be caused by a so-called exogenous
virus. In free-roaming cats, feline leukaemia virus seems to be wide-
spread, since many cats have antibodies to a virus-associated antigen
(Jarrett, 1976). However, leukaemia is a relatively rare disease in these
animals. This indicates that host factors strongly control the development of the disease.

  With regard to the avian leukosis viruses resistance to the different
viral subgroups is controlled by single recessive genes and can be
explained by lack of the appropriate receptors (Piraino, 1967).
Probably multiple alleles occur at the various loci as different levels of

resistance can be encountered (Payne, 1972). Whereas resistance to avain leukosis viruses usually is recessive, single instances of dominance have been found (Payne, 1972). Probably a completely different physiological mechanism and not lack of receptors underlies this resistance.

Receptors have been shown to be important for mammalian oncoviruses (deLarco and Todaro, 1976) but genetic polymorphism within a species with regard to the presence of such receptors has not yet been found. A locus *Fv-1* has been described in mice by Lilly and Pincus (1973), which controls tropism of murine leukaemia viruses. Resistance induced by this locus for one type virus proves to be a dominant trait. The heterozygote is not only refractory to one type of virus but also to the alternate category. The well-known laboratory strains of MuLV, like Rauscher virus, escape control by this locus. There are some indications that the gene product of *Fv-1* interferes with the transcription of proviral DNA after integration into the host genome (Jollicoeur and Baltimore, 1976).

The *Fv-1* gene has first been described in relation to the genetics of susceptibility to the induction of foci of transformed erythroblasts in the spleen by the Friends strain of MuLV (Lilly, 1970). Another gene, *Fv-2*, was also described which probably controls an intrinsic property of the erythroid compartment to become transformed. Possibly the *Fv-2* gene interferes with the *onc*-gene of this virus strain.

In the MuMTV system, in which resistance proves to be recessive (Bentvelzen et al., 1972), a good correlation has been found between genetic susceptibility and replication of the virus (Mühlbock, 1956; Hairstone et al., 1964). This suggests that a higher rate of transcription of the provirus, leading to an increased number of 35S molecular, also results in a higher number of messages from the *onc*-gene (called *mam* by Hilgers and Bentvelzen, 1978). It cannot be excluded, however, that the control would be at the translational level.

Immunosurveillance seems to play an important role in the control of virus-induced neoplasia in cats (Essex and Lamon, 1976). It can be imagined that genes controlling immunological responses to feline leukaemia virus play a definite role in the suppression of the disease. Such genes remain to be detected, however.

The role of the *H-2* gene in viral leukemogenesis in mice (see Démant and Cleton in this volume) might be ascribed to an immunological response to the virus. *H-2* controlled resistance to viral leukaemogenesis is associated with high titers of antibodies to the viral envelope (Nowinski et al., 1976; Tucker et al., 1977; Bubbers et al., 1977; Melief et al., 1978). An alternative explanation is that *H-2* con-

trolled excessive virus replication leads to immunological unrespon-
siveness to the virus.

In the rat strain differences have been found in antibody response
to MuLV proteins. The major histocompatibility locus *AgB* seems to
be associated with these differences, although other loci also seem to
be involved (Jones et al., 1978). The rat strain BN with the highest
antibody titer, also replicates the virus best and is the most susceptible to its oncogenic action. These results would suggest antibody response of no relevance to the suppression of the disease.

In the MuMTV system the resistance of the I mouse strain to the
virus is most likely due to a good cellular immunological response to
virally transformed cells (Nandi et al., 1972).

In conclusion, genetical factors have been described in various
oncovirus systems which interfere with several aspects of the life
cycle of these viruses, impeding the cancerous process. Several other
host genes have been described which have an affect on the disease
(Heston, 1963; Lilly and Pincus, 1973), but often they mediate their
action through an effect on growth rate in general.

6. ENDOGENOUS RNA TUMOUR VIRUSES

In his classical review on lysogeny, Lwoff (1953) suggested that
lysogeny could have its animal counterpart in carcinogenesis. Lwoff
(1960) detailed this supposition in showing that neoplasia could result
from either the integration of the genome of an exogenous virus or the
induction of genetically transmitted endogenous viruses.

Moore (1963) suggested lysogeny could play a role in the MuMTV
system: it might explain the seemingly aberrant transmission of the
late-oncogenic MuMTV variant in the C3Hf strain. Law (1966) suggested that the leukaemia virus in AKR mice might be transmitted genetically from parents to offspring.

The hypothesis of genetic transmission got impetus by the genetical
study on gamete-born transmission of MuMTV in the GR strain
(Bentvelzen, 1968; Bentvelzen and Daams, 1969; Bentvelzen et al.,
1970). Subsequent studies led to the hypothesis that every mouse
strain would contain genetic information for a MuMTV in its normal
cellular DNA. Usually transcription of such a germinal provirus would
be repressed, but either due to mutations in controlling genes or to
temporary abrogation of repression by carcinogenic treatment, virus
would be released.

The following observations support this hypothesis.

1. Introduction of a virus which is transmitted by the gametes in a given mouse strain into another mouse strain only leads to milkborne transmission (Mühlbock and Bentvelzen, 1968).

2. In various crosses virus release seems to be controlled by a single dominant gene (Bentvelzen, 1968; 1972; Mühlbock and Bentvelzen, 1968; Bentvelzen and Daams, 1969; van Nie et al., 1972; 1975; 1976; 1977).

3. Virus (Timmermans et al., 1969) or viral footprints (Bentvelzen, 1972; Schlom et al., 1973) can be induced in mice of low-cancer strains by carcinogenic treatments.

4. Virus (Hageman et al., 1972; Bentvelzen, 1975) or viral footprints (Bentvelzen, 1972) can be found in old mice of low-cancer-strain mice, even when they are kept in a germ-free condition (Bentvelzen, 1975).

5. Virus can be induced in kidney culture of low-cancer-strain mice by methylcholanthrene (Links et al., 1972), glucocorticoids (Bentvelzen, 1974b) or halogenated pyrimidines (Bentvelzen, 1975).

6. Molecular hybridization studies reveal that normal cellular DNA of every mouse strain tested so far contains multiple copies of the MuMTV genome (Scolnick et al., 1974; Morris et al., 1977).

In the case of the virulent MuMTV-P in the GR mouse strain, virus release is associated with rapid tumour development. With regard to the late-oncogenic MuMTV-strains, considerable evidence has been obtained for an increased risk of tumour development in animals releasing virus, but also tumours come up in so-called virus-free animals (Van Nie et al., 1975; Bentvelzen et al., 1978).

The release of the virulent MuMTV-P in the GR mouse strain, controlled by a single dominant gene, is not impeded by genetic factors from any mouse strain tested so far. Only minor effects upon tumour age have been described (Bentvelzen and Daams, 1969; Van Nie and Hilgers, 1976).

In crosses between the C3Hf mouse strain, which spontaneously releases a late-oncogenic MuMTV, and the mouse strain BALB/c, which does not release virus, the expression of MuMTV seems to be controlled by a single dominant gene *Mtv-1* (Van Nie et al., 1975). The inhibition of virus-release in the BALB/c strain does not affect that of MuMTV-L from C3Hf. Reciprocally, the *Mtv-1* gene cannot induce release of virulent virus carried by the BALB/c strain. The various controlling elements are concerned with only their own provirus, to which they are probably closely linked. Some mouse strains like C57BL carry a dominant epistatic gene *Imv*, which inhibits MuMTV-L expression in hybrid with C3Hf to a large extent (Bentvelzen et al., 1978).

In the GR mouse strain besides the gene *Mtv-2*, which causes the uninhibited release of a virulent MuMTV, there seem also to be other genes which cause the release of considerably lesser oncogenic viruses, which cause tumours at a late age (Bentvelzen, 1974b; Bentvelzen et al., in press).

Inhibition of virus expression can be due in some mouse strains like BALB/c to absence of transcription of the MuMTV proviruses; in others like C57BL transcription takes place but no MuMTV proteins are formed, indicating repression at the translational level (Michalides et al., 1978).

At the same time, when the genetic transmission theory of MuMTV was developed, Huebner and Todaro (1969) launched the virogene-oncogene hypothesis, which claims that every vertebrate would carry genetic information (virogene) for a C-type oncovirus, and that a single gene (oncogene) of this virogene would control neoplastic conversion in every tissue, irrespective of the initial carcinogenic stimulus. Indeed in many different animal species multiple germinal proviruses of type-C viruses have been found (Todaro, 1978), but in most instances oncogenic potential of these endogenous viruses remains to be established.

In the AKR mouse strain early T-cell leukaemia seems to be a hereditary trait, but also virally induced (Gross, 1970). It has recently been demonstrated that neoplastic conversion of thymic cells is induced by a novel type virus, which results from the recombination of an endogenous virus, which is released at an early age and grows well in mouse cells (*ecotropic*), with another endogenous C-type oncovirus, which cannot grow in mouse cells (*xenotropic*) and which is released at a late age (Hartley et al., 1977). The leukaemia would result from the integration of a somatic provirus of the recombinant virus (Figure 5). Such recombination events in the generation of new highly oncogenic viruses seems to be a far more common event than previously realized (Rapp et al., 1978).

The recombination hypothesis has the danger of becoming a doctrine. In the breeding colony of our institute a recessive mutation arose in a line of the C3Hf strain, which led to the early development of leukaemia (before 3 months of age). These leukaemias produce C-type oncovirus abundantly (K. Nooter, unpublished results); bioassays of the virus are still underway. The mutation probably took place in a dominant epistatic inhibitory gene, comparable to the *Imv* gene in the MuMTV-system and the I^e gene, controlling expression of endogenous

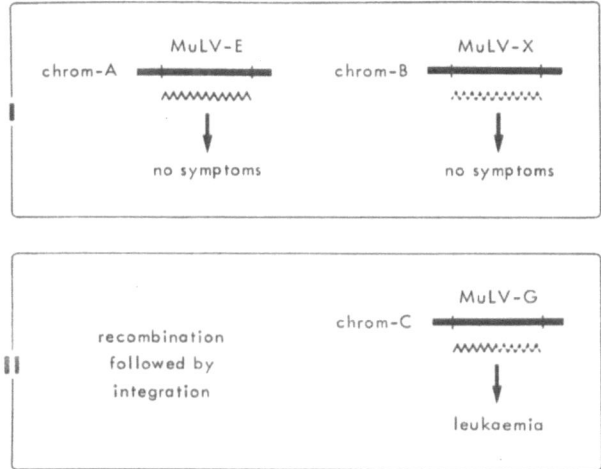

Figure 5. Generation of an oncogenic tumour virus by recombination of endogenous viruses of which one is ecotropic (E) and the other xenotropic (X).

avian C-type oncovirus (Payne, 1972). Since no increase in proviral copies on leukaemic cell DNA can be found as compared to normal liver DNA (K.J. van den Berg, unpublished results), it is unlikely that in this subline recombinant viruses would be involved in the leukaemogenic process.

There is also no indication in the GR mouse strain that the induction of mammary tumours is due to integration of an additional provirus (Michalides et al., 1976).

As stated above the oncogenic activity of many endogenous C-type oncoviruses remains to be established. A handicap is that many of these viruses cannot replicate in cells of their own species. However, the aforementioned recombination story indicates that such viruses may carry an *onc*-gene. Continuous expression of such viruses, or of at least their *onc-gene*, may result in neoplastic conversion. I do not think that one and the same *onc*-gene of such endogenous viruses would cause tumours in every tissue.

ACKNOWLEDGEMENTS

Reported studies in our own laboratory have been supported by the Koningin Wilhelmina Fonds, the Netherlands Organization for the Fight against Cancer, and the U.S. National Cancer Institute, Virus Cancer Program (Contract No. 1 CP4-3328).

REFERENCES

Aaronson, S.A. (1973). Biologic characterization of mammalian cells transformed by a primate sarcoma virus. Virology 52: 562-567.
Axel, R., J. Schlom and S. Spiegelman (1972). Presence in human breast cancer RNA homologous to mouse mammary tumour virus RNA. Nature 235: 32-36.
Baltimore, D. (1970). Viral RNA-dependent DNA polymerase. Nature 226: 1209-1211.
Baltimore, D. (1975). Tumor Viruses: 1974. Cold Spring Harbor Symp. Quant. Biol. 39: 1187-1200.
Bentvelzen, P. (1968). Genetical control of the vertical transmission of the Mühlbock mammary tumour virus in the GR mouse strain. Hollandia, Amsterdam.
Bentvelzen, P. (1972). Hereditary infections with mammary tumor viruses in mice. In "RNA Viruses and Host Genome in Oncogenesis", P. Emmelot and P. Bentvelzen, eds., North-Holland, Amsterdam, pp. 309-337.
Bentvelzen, P. (1974a). Comparative biology of murine and avian tumor viruses. In "Viruses, Evolution and Cancer", E. Kurstak and K. Maramorosch, eds., Academic Press, New York, pp. 280-367.
Bentvelzen, P. (1974b). Host-virus interaction in murine mammary carcinogenesis. Biochim. Biophys. Acta 355: 236-259.
Bentvelzen, P. (1975). Endogenous mammary tumor viruses in mice. Cold Spring Harbor Symp. Quart. Biol. 39: 1145-1151.
Bentvelzen, P. and J. Brinkhof (1977). Organ distribution of exogenous murine mammary tumour virus as determined by bioassay. Europ. J. Cancer 13: 241-246.
Bentvelzen, P. and P.C. Creemers (1977). Natural immunity to murine mammary tumor viruses. In "Contemporary topics in immunobiology", M.G. Hanna Jr. and F. Rapp, eds., Vol. 6, Plenum, New York, pp. 229-238.
Bentvelzen, P. and J.H. Daams (1969). Hereditary infections with mammary tumor viruses in mice. J. Natl. Cancer Inst. 43: 1025-1035.
Bentvelzen, P., J. Brinkhof, and J.J. Haaijman (1978). Genetic control of the release of endogenous murine mammary tumour viruses reinvestigated. Europ. J. Cancer 14: 1137-1147.
Bentvelzen, P., J.H. Daams, P. Hageman and J. Calafat (1970). Genetic transmission of viruses that incite mammary tumor in mice. Proc. Natl. Acad. Sci. USA 67: 377-384.
Bentvelzen, P., J.H. Daams, P. Hageman, J. Calafat and A. Timmermans (1972). Interactions between viral and genetic factors in the origin of mammary tumors in mice. J. Natl. Cancer Inst. 48: 1089-1094.
Bergholz, C.M., L.G. Wolfe, F. Deinhardt, B. Thakkar and B. Marczynska (1977). Oncogenicity in marmosets of HL-23V, a type-C oncornavirus isolated from human leukemic cells, and comparison with simian sarcomavirus type 1 (SSV-1/ SSAV-1). J. Natl. Cancer Inst. 58: 1041-1046.
Bernhard, W. (1958). Electron microscopy of tumor cells and tumor viruses: A review. Cancer Res. 18: 491-509.
Black, M.M., R.E. Zachrav, B. Shore, A.S. Dion and H.P. Leis, Jr. (1975). Cellular immunity to autologous breast cancer and RIII-murine mammary tumor virus preparations. Cancer Res. 38: 2068-2076.
Bolognesi, D.P., R.C. Montelaro, H. Frank and W. Schäfer (1978). Assembly of type-C oncornaviruses: A model. Science 199: 183-186.
Brommer, E.J.P. and P. Bentvelzen (1974). The haemopoietic stem cell in Rauscher virus-induced erythroblastosis of BALB/c mice. Europ. J. Cancer 10: 827-833.
Brugge, J. and R. Erikson (1977). Identification of a transformation-specific antigen induced by an avian sarcoma virus. Nature 269:346-348.

Bubbers, J.E., K.J. Blank, H.A. Freedman and F. Lilly (1977). Mechanisms of the H-2 effect on viral leukemogenesis. Scand. J. Immunol. 6: 533-538.

Cardiff, R.D., M.J. Puentes, Y.A. Teramoto and J.K, Lund (1974). Structure of the mouse mammary tumor virus: Characterization of bald particles. J. Virol. 14: 1293-1303.

Cohen, J.C., P.R. Shank, R. Cardiff and H.E. Varmus (1978). Analysis of the proviruses of mouse mammary tumor viruses endogenous to normal mice and acquired during infection in vivo. 11th Meeting on Mammary Cancer in Experimental Animals and Man. Detroit, Abstr. p. 90.

Collett, M.S. and R.L. Erikson (1978). Protein kinase activity associated with the avian sarcoma virus src gene product. Proc. Natl. Acad. Sci. USA 75: 2021-2024.

Cunningham-Rundles, S., W.F. Feller, C. Cunningham-Rundles, B. Dupont, H. Wanebo, R. O'Reilly and R.A. Good (1976). Lymphocyte transformation in vitro to RIII mouse milk antigen among women with breast disease. Cell. Immunol. 25: 322-327.

De Larco, J. and G.J. Todaro (1976). Membrane receptors for murine leukaemia viruses: characterization using the purified viral envelope glycoprotein, gp71. Cell 8: 365-372.

Duesberg, P., P.K. Vogt, K. Beemon and M. Lai (1975). Avian RNA tumor viruses: Mechanism of recombination and complexity of the genome. Cold Spring Harbor Symp. Quart. Biol. 39: 847-858.

Essex, M. and E.W. Lamon (1975). Host immune response to oncornavirus-induced tumors. In "Comparative Leukemia Research 1975", J. Clemmesen and D.S. Yohn, eds., Karger, Basel, pp. 166-172.

Fenner, F. (1976). The classification and nomenclature of viruses. September 1978. Acta Virol. 20: 170-181.

Fenyö, E.M., E. Yefenof and G. Klein (1977). Immunization of mice with syngeneic Moloney lymphoma cells induces separate antibodies against virion envelope glycoprotein and virus-induced cell surface antigens. J. Exp. Med. 146: 1521-1533.

Gallagher, R.E. and R.C. Gallo (1975). Type-C RNA tumor virus isolated from cultured human acute myelogenous leukemia cells. Science 187: 350-353.

Gielkens, A.L.J., D. van Zaane, H.P.J. Bloemers and H. Bloemendal (1976). Synthesis of Rauscher murine leukemia virus specific polypeptides in vitro. Proc. Natl. Acad. Sci. USA 73: 356-360.

Graf, T. (1973). In vitro transformation of chicken bone marrow cells with avian erythroblastosis virus. Z. Naturforsch. 30: 847-848, 1975.

Gross, L. (1970). Oncogenic Viruses. Oxford, Pergamon Press.

Hairstone, M.A., J.B. Sheffield and D.H. Moore (1964). Study of B-particles in mammary tumors of different mouse strains. J. Natl. Cancer Inst. 33: 825-836.

Hageman, P., J. Calafat and J.H. Daams (1972). The mouse mammary tumor viruses. In "RNA Viruses and Host Genome in Oncogenesis", P. Emmelot and P. Bentvelzen, eds., Amsterdam, North-Holland, pp. 283-300.

Hanafusa, H., T. Hanafusa and H. Rubin (1963). The defectiveness of Rous sarcoma virus. Proc. Natl. Acad. Sci. USA 49: 572-580.

Hartley, J.W. and W.P. Rowe (1966). Production of altered cell foci in tissue culture by defective Moloney sarcoma virus particles Proc. Natl. Acad. Sci. USA 55: 780-786.

Hartley, J.W., N.K. Wolford, L.J. Old and W.P. Rowe (1977). A new class of murine leukemia virus associated with development of spontaneous lymphomas. Proc. Natl. Acad. Sci. USA 74: 789-792.

Heston, W.E. (1963). Genetics of neoplasia. In "Methodology in Mammalian Genetics", W.J. Burdette, ed., Holden Day, San Francisco, pp. 247-268.

Hilgers, J. and P. Bentvelzen (1978). Interaction between viral and genetic factors in murine mammary cancer. Adv. Cancer Research 26: 143-195.

Huebner, R.J. and G.J. Todaro (1969). Oncogenes of RNA tumor viruses as determinants of cancer. Proc. Natl. Acad. Sci. USA 64: 1087-1091.

Jarrett, W.F.H. (1976). The epidemiology of feline leukemia virus infection. In "Comparative Leukemia Research 1975", J. Clemmesen and D.S. Yohn, eds., pp. 209-211.

Jolicoeur, P. and D. Baltimore (1976). Effect of *Fv-1* gene product on synthesis of N-tropic and B-tropic murine leukemia viral RNA. Cell 7: 33-39.

Jones, J.M., F. Jensen and J.D. Feldman (1978). Genetic control of immune responses to Moloney leukemia virus in rats. J. Natl. Cancer Inst. 60: 1467-1472.

Karshin, W.L., L.J. Arcement, R.B. Naso and R.B. Arlinghaus (1977). Common precursor for Rauscher leukemia virus for gp69/71, p15E and p12E. J. Virol. 23: 787-798.

Kopchik, J.J., G.A. Jamjoon, K.F. Watson and R.B. Arlinghaus (1978). Biosynthesis of reverse transcriptase from Rauscher murine leukemia virus by synthesis and cleavage of a gag-pol read-through viral precursor polyprotein. Proc. Nat. Acad. Sci. USA 75: 2016-2020.

Kung, H.J., J.M. Baily, N. Davidson, M.O. Nicolson and R.M. McAllister (1975). Structure, subunit composition, and molecular weight of RD-114 RNA. J. Virol. 16: 397-411.

Kurth, R. and G. Kitchener (1978). Tumor antigen induction by the envelope-defective Bryan strain of Rous sarcoma virus. J. Natl. Cancer Inst. 60: 1365-1369.

Langlois, A.J., D. Beard and J.W. Beard (1970). Strain MC29, an avian leukosis virus of unique properties. Bibl. Haematol. 36: 96-105.

Law, L.W. (1966). Transmission studies of a leukemogenic virus, MLV, in mice. Natl. Cancer Inst. Monogr. 22: 267-285.

Lilly, F. (1970). *Fv-2*: Identification and location of a second gene governing the spleen focus response to Friend leukemia virus in mice. J. Natl. Cancer Inst. 45: 163-169.

Lilly, F. and T. Pincus (1973). Genetic control of murine viral leukemogenesis. Adv. Cancer Res. 17: 231-277.

Links, J., F. Buijs and O. Tol (1972). In vitro transformation of baby mouse kidney cells with the mouse mammary tumour virus. In "Fundamental Research on Mammary Tumours," J. Mouriquand, ed., Inserm, Paris, pp. 263-268.

Lwoff, A. (1953). Lysogeny, Bacteriol. Rev. 17: 269-337.

Lwoff, A. (1960). Tumor viruses and the cancer problem: A summation of the conference. Cancer Res. 20: 820-829.

Melief, C.J., A. Vlug, W. Barendsen, C. de Bruijne and T.L. Molenaar (1978). Ecotropic type C RNA virus expression and its consequences in congenic resistant C57BL mice. In "Advances in Comparative Leukemia Research 1977," P. Bentvelzen, J. Hilgers and D.S. Yohn, eds., Elsevier/North-Holland, Amsterdam, pp. 78-83.

Mesa-Tejada, R., I. Keydar, M. Ramanarayanan, T. Ohno, C. Fenoglio and S. Spiegelman (1978). Detection in human breast carcinomas of an antigen immunologically related to a group-specific antigen of mouse mammary tumor virus. Proc. Natl. Acad. Sci. USA 75: 1529-1533.

Michalides, R. and R. Nusse (1978). Factors influencing the expression of the endogenous MuMTV. 11th Meeting on Mammary Cancer in Experimental Animals and Man. Detroit, Abstr. p. 24.

Michalides, R., G. Vlahakis and J. Schlom (1976). A biochemical approach to the study of the transmission of mouse mammary tumor viruses in mouse strains RIII and C3H. Int. J. Cancer 18: 105-115.

Michalides, R., L. van Deemter and R. van Nie (1978). Identification of the *Mtv-2* gene responsible for the early appearance of mammary tumors in the GR mouse by nucleic acid hybridization. Proc. Natl. Acad. Sci. USA 75: 2368-2372.

Moore, D.H. (1963). Mouse mammary tumour agent and mouse mammary tumours. Nature 198: 429-433.

Morris, V.L., E. Medeiros, G.M. Ringold, J.M. Bishop and H.E. Varmus (1977). Comparison of mouse mammary tumor virus-specific DNA in inbred, wild and Asian mice, and in tumors and normal organs from inbred mice. J. Mol. Biol. 114: 73-91.

Mühlbock, O. (1956). Biological studies on the mammary tumor agent in different strains of mice. Acta Unio Int. contra Cancrum 12: 665-681.

Mühlbock, O. and P. Bentvelzen (1968). The transmission of the mammary tumor viruses. In "Perspectives in Virology," Vol. 6, M. Pollard, ed., Academic Press, New York, pp. 75-87.

Müller, M., S. Zotter and C. Kemmer (1976). Specificity of human antibodies to intracytoplasmic type-A particles of murine mammary tumor virus. J. Natl. Cancer Inst. 56: 295-303.

Nandi, S., S. Haslam and C. Helmich (1972). Mechanisms of resistance to mammary tumor development in C57BL and I strains of mice. I. Noduligenesis, tumorigenesis, and characteristics of nodules and tumors. J. Natl. Cancer Inst. 48: 1005-1012.

Naso, R.B., L.J. Arcement and R.B. Arlinghaus (1975). Biosynthesis of Rauscher leukemia viral proteins. Cell 4: 31-36.

Nie, R. van and J. Hilgers (1976). Genetic analysis of mammary tumor induction and expression of mammary tumor virus antigen in hormone-treated ovariectomized GR mice. J. Natl. Cancer Inst. 56: 27-32.

Nie, R. van and A.A. Verstraeten (1975). Studies of genetic transmission of mammary tumor virus by C3Hf mice. Int. J. Cancer 16: 922-931.

Nie, R. van, J. Hilgers and M. Lenselink (1972). Genetical analysis of mammary tumour development and mammary tumour virus expression in the GR mouse. In "Fundamental Research on Mammary Tumours," J. Mouriquand, ed., Inserm. Paris, pp. 21-30.

Nie, R. van, A.A. Verstraeten and J. de Moes (1977). Genetic transmission of mammary tumour virus by GR mice. Int. J. Cancer 19: 383-390.

Nooter, K. and P. Bentvelzen (1977). *In vitro* transformation by RNA tumor viruses. In "Recent advances in cancer research: Cell biology, molecular biology, and tumor virology," Vol. 1, R.C. Gallo, ed., CRC Press, Cleveland, pp. 175-188.

Nooter, K., A.M. Aarssen, P. Bentvelzen, F.G. de Groot and F.G. van Pelt (1975). Isolation of infectious C-type oncornavirus from human leukaemic bone marrow cells. Nature 256: 595-597.

Nooter, K., P. Bentvelzen, C. Zurcher and J. Rhim (1977). Detection of human C-type "helper" viruses in human leukemic bone marrow with murine sarcoma virus-transformed human and rat non-producer cells. Int. J. Cancer 19: 59-65.

Nooter, K., J., Overdevest, R. Dubbes, G. Koch, P. Bentvelzen, C. Zurcher, J. Coolen and J. Calafat (1978). Type-C oncovirus isolated from human leukemic bone marrow: Further *in vitro* and *in vivo* characterization. Int. J. Cancer 21: 27-34.

Nowinski, R.C. and T. Doyle (1976). Antibody to murine leukemia virus: Genetic control linked to the H-2 locus in BL mice. J. Immunol. 117: 350-351.

Oppermann, H., J.M. Bishop, H.E. Varmus and L. Levintow (1977). A joint product of the genes *gag* and *pol* of avian sarcoma virus: a possible precursor of reverse transcriptase. Cell 12: 993-1005.

Payne, L.N. (1972). Interactions between host genome and avian RNA tumor viruses. In "RNA Viruses and Host Genome in Oncogenesis," P. Emmelot and P. Bentvelzen, eds., North-Holland, Amsterdam, pp. 93-115.

Piraino, F. (1967). The mechanism of genetic resistance of chick embryo cells to infection by Rous sarcoma virus-Bryan strain (BS-RSV). Virology 32: 700-707.

Rapp, K.R. and G.J. Todaro (1978). Generation of oncogenic type C viruses: Rapidly leukemogenic viruses derived from C3H mouse cells *in vivo* and *in vitro*. Proc. Natl. Acad. Sci. USA 75: 2468-2472.

Schidlovsky, G. (1977). Structure of RNA tumor viruses. In "Recent Advances in Cancer Research: Cell Biology, Molecular Biology, and Tumor Virology," Vol. 1, R.C. Gallo, ed., CRC Press, Cleveland, pp. 189-245.

Schlom, J., R. Michalides, D. Kufe, R. Hehlmann, S. Spiegelman, P. Bentvelzen and P. Hageman (1973). A comparative study of the biologic and molecular basis of murine mammary carcinoma: A model for human breast cancer. J. Natl. Cancer Inst. 51: 541-551.

Scolnick, E.M., W.P. Parks, T. Kawakami, D. Kohne, H. Okabe, R.V. Gilden and M. Hatanaka (1974). Primate and murine type-C viral nucleic acid association kinetics: Analysis of model systems and natural tissues. J. Virol. 13: 363-369.

Snyder, H.W. Jr., E. Stockert and E. Fleissner (1977). Characterization of the molecular species carrying Gross cell surface antigen. J. Virol. 23: 302-314.

Stephenson, J.R., S.R. Tronick and S.A. Aaronson (1975). Murine leukemia virus mutants with temperature-sensitive defects in precursor polypeptide cleavage. Cell 6: 543-550.

Stephenson, J.R., M. Essex, S. Hino, W.D. Hardy, Jr. and S.A. Aaronson (1977). Feline oncornavirus-associated membrane antigen (FOCMA). VII. Distinction between FOCMA and the major virion glycoprotein. Proc. Nat. Acad. Sci. USA 74: 1219-1223.

Svoboda, J. and I. Hložánek (1970). Role of cell association in virus infection and virus rescue. Adv. Cancer Res. 13: 217-269.

Temin, H.M. and S. Mizutani (1970). RNA-dependent DNA polymerase in virions of Rous sarcoma virus. Nature 226: 1211-1213.

Timmermans, A., P. Bentvelzen, P.C. Hageman and J. Calafat (1969). Activation of a mammary tumour virus in 020 strain mice by X-irradiation and urethane. J. Gen. Virol. 4: 619-621.

Todaro, G.J. (1978). RNA-tumour-virus genes and transforming genes: Patterns of transmission. British J. Cancer 37: 139-158.

Tooze, J. (1973). The molecular biology of tumor viruses. Cold Spring Harbor Laboratory, New York.

Tucker, H.S.G., J. Weens, P. Tsichlis, R.S. Schwartz, R. Khiroya and J. Donnelly (1977). Influence of H-2 complex on susceptibility to infection by murine leukemia virus. J. Immunol. 118: 1239-1243.

Varmus, H.E., J. Stavnezer, E. Medeiros and J.M. Bishop (1975). Detection and characterization of RNA tumor virus-specific DNA in cells. In "Comparative Leukemia Research 1973," Y. Ito and R.M. Dutcher, eds., Leukemogenesis. University of Tokyo Press. pp. 451-461.

Weissmann, C., J.T. Parsons, J.W. Coffin, L. Rymo, M.A. Billeter and H. Hofstetter (1975). Studies on the structure and synthesis of Rous sarcoma virus RNA. Cold Spring Harbor Symp. Quart. Biol. 39: 1043-1056.

Westenbrink, F., W. Koornstra and P. Bentvelzen (1977). The major polypeptides of the murine mammary tumour virus isolated by plantlectin affinity chromatography. Europ. J. Biochem. 76: 85-90.

Westenbrink, F., W. Koornstra, J. Brinkhof, P. Creemers and P. Bentvelzen (1979). Cellular localization of the major polypeptides of the murine mammary tumour virus. Europ. J. Cancer 15: 109-121.

Witte, D.N. and D. Baltimore (1978). Relationship of retrovirus polyprotein cleavages to virion maturation studied with temperature sensitive murine leukemia virus mutants. J. Virol. 26: 750-761.

Wu, A.M. (1967). The biochemical life cycle of type C RNA tumor viruses. In "Recent Advances in Cancer Research: Cell Biology, Molecular Biology, and Tumor Virology," Vol. II, R.C. Gallo, ed., CRC Press, Cleveland, pp. 1-36.

Yeger, H., V.I. Kalnins and J.R. Stephenson (1976). Electron microscopy of mammalian type C RNA viruses: Use of conditional lethal mutants in studies of virion maturation and assembly. Virology 74: 459-469.

Zaane, D. van, A.L.J. Gielkens, M.J.A. Dekker-Michielsen and H.P.J. Bloemers (1975). Virus-specific precursor polypeptides in cells infected with Rauscher leukemia virus. Virology 67: 544-552.

Zaane, D. van, A.L.J. Gielkens, W.G. Hesselink and H.P.J. Bloemers (1977). Identification of Rauscher murine leukemia virus-specific mRNAs for the synthesis of gag- and env-gene products. Proc. Natl. Acad. Sci. USA 74: 1855-1859.

5. STRUCTURE AND FUNCTIONS OF ADENOVIRUS 5 TRANSFORMATION GENES

A.J. VAN DER EB, H. JOCHEMSEN, J.H. LUPKER, J. MAAT, H. VAN ORMONDT and P.I. SCHRIER

ABSTRACT

Transformation by human adenoviruses is a process in which only a small part of the genome is involved. The transforming segment is localized at the left-hand end of the genome, between 1 and 11%, corresponding to the early region 1.

Transformation studies with DNA fragments of non-oncogenic adenovirus 5 have shown that, in addition to fragments containing the entire left-hand early region, smaller fragments representing various parts of this early region also contain transforming activity. When the properties of baby rat kidney lines transformed by fragments of various sizes were compared, it was observed that the cell lines were not identical in their properties but could be divided into at least 3 categories: (1) cells transformed by the entire left-hand early region (0-11%); (2) cells transformed by the *Hind*III (*Hsu*I) G fragment (0-8%); and (3) cells transformed by the *Hpa*I E fragment (0-4.5%).

This suggested that transformation by adenovirus 5 is a process in which more than one viral gene is involved. Experiments to identify these genes and their protein products are described, using in vitro protein synthesis, immunoprecipitation and nucleotide sequence analysis. It was found that the left-hand 4.5% of the genome (fragmen *Hpa*I E) codes for a series of (partially) overlapping proteins, which apparently have the ability to transform a diploid cell with a limited life span into a permanent cell line. The adjacent segment (4.5-9 or 11%) codes for at least 2 major proteins which apparently are responsible for the induction of a number of properties that are characteristic for transformed cells.

Many lines of evidence suggest that only part of the genome of DNA and RNA tumor viruses is involved in the process of cell transformation. The most convincing proof for this suggestion is the finding that specific fragments of the DNA from some tumor viruses are able to

F.J. Cleton and J.W.I.M. Simons (eds.), Genetic Origins of Tumor Cells. 73–85.
Copyright © 1980 by Martinus Nijhoff Publishers bv, The Hague/Boston/London.
All rights reserved.

cause transformation in vitro, and in some cases, induce tumors in animals.

This paper presents a summary of the work carried out in our laboratory on the identification and characterization of the genes of human adenoviruses involved in transformation.

In 1973 a new technique, the "Calcium" or "Calcium-phosphate" technique, was developed in our laboratory by Dr. F.L. Graham which made possible the transformation of cells in culture with DNA from adenoviruses and from other DNA tumorviruses (SV40, BK virus, Herpes simplex virus (c.f. Graham and Van der Eb, 1973a, b; Abrahams and Van der Eb, 1975; Van der Noordaa, 1976; Bacchetti and Graham, 1977). Further experiments indicated that the infectivity (i.e. the ability to produce infectious progeny virus) was lost when the viral DNA was broken into fragments, but that the transforming activity was not inactivated and remained unchanged, provided that the fragments did not become too small (Graham et al., 1974a, b). This indicated that the integrity of the viral genome is not required for transformation, and it also suggested that only a fraction of the genome is involved in this process. Further studies with viral DNA fragments obtained by cleavage with restriction endonucleases unequivocally confirmed this conclusion, and demonstrated that the transforming activity is localized in a relatively small segment of the viral DNA in all adenovirus serotypes tested so far (Graham et al., 1974; Van der Eb et al., 1977; Van der Eb and Houweling, 1977). Figure 1 shows a summary of the restriction enzyme fragments of adenovirus 5 (Ad5) DNA that were found to contain transforming

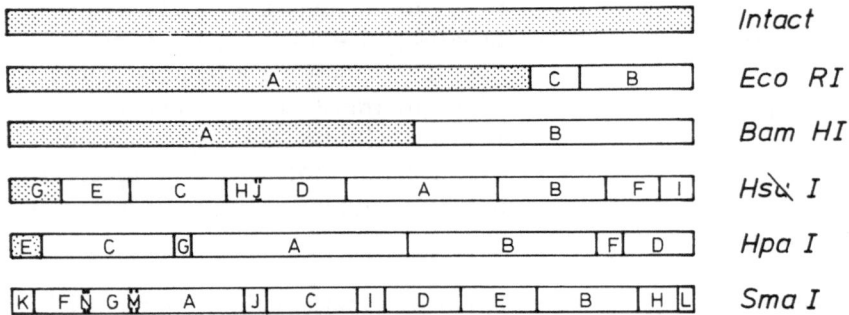

Figure 1. Maps of adenovirus 5 DNA showing the cleavage sites of a number of restriction endonucleases (endo R.). The shaded fragments were found to contain transforming activity. The *Eco*RI and *Hpa*I maps are taken from Mulder et al. (1974), and the *Bam*HI, *Hsu*I and *Sma*I maps from Mulder and Greene (personal communication).

activity. It can be seen that all transforming fragments are located in the left part of the DNA and that transformation was still obtained with very small fragments.

When we compared the properties of a series of baby rat kidney cells transformed by Ad5 DNA fragments of various sizes, we observed that these cells were not identical in properties but could be divided roughly into 3 categories:

1. Cells transformed by the larger DNA fragments (*Eco* RI A, *Bam* HI A). These cells contain the entire left-hand early region, which maps between 1 and 11%; we have called these cells the "standard" transformed cells.
2. Cells transformed by the 8% *Hsu* I G fragment. These cells contain most of the left-hand early region, but lack the area between 8 and 11%.
3. Cells transformed by the 4.5% *Hpa*I E fragment, which contain less than half of the leftmost early region.

Table 1. Properties of baby rat kidney cells transformed by left-end fragments of adenovirus 5 DNA.

DNA in transformed cells	Lifespan	Karyotype	Saturation density (monolayer)	Cell morphology	T antigen (IF)
⩾ 11%	unlimited	aneuploid	high	epithelial	typical
8% *Hsu*I G	unlimited	aneuploid	high	epithelial	atypical
4.5% *Hpa*I E	unlimited	aneuploid	low	± fibro-blastic	atypical

The differences between the 3 categories of transformed cells are summarized in Table I. It can be seen that the *Hsu* I G-transformed cells have a normal transformed phenotype. When the T antigen was studied by immunofluorescence, however, it was found that all G fragment-transformed cells had an atypical distribution of T antigen, in that it was localized predominantly in the cytoplasm rather than in the nucleus (see Figure 2). In addition, the concentration of T antigen appeared to be lower in G fragment-transformed than in the standard transformed cells.

The cells in the third category, transformed by the 4.5% *Hpa*I E fragment, are also characterized by an atypical (cytoplasmic) distribution of T antigen (their T antigen concentration is even lower than in the G-fragment transformed cells). E fragment-transformed cells differ, however, from cells transformed by larger fragments in a number of other phenotypical properties: first, the cells grow more slowly,

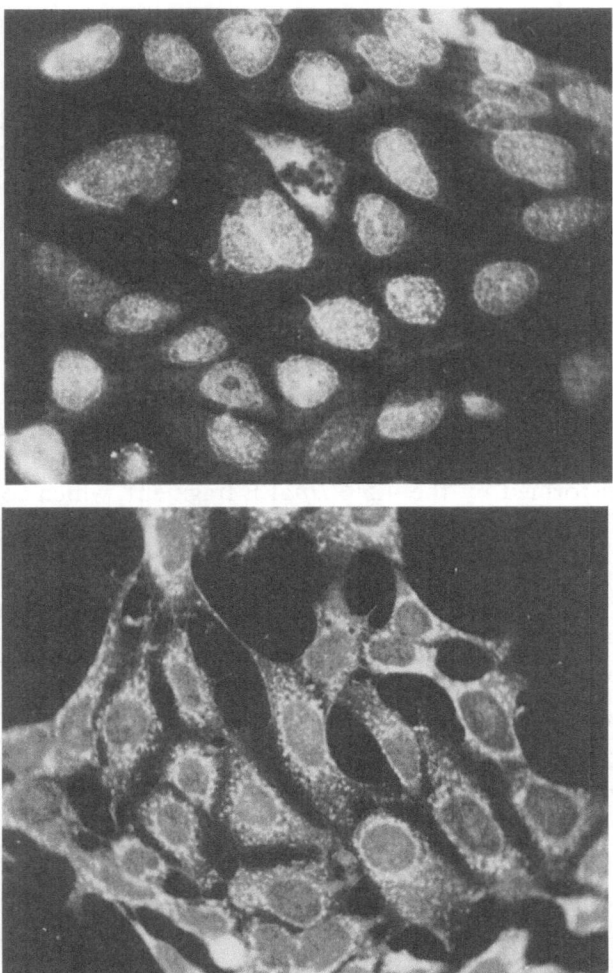

Figure 2. Immunofluorescence of virus-specific T antigen in baby rat kidney (BRK) cells transformed by adenovirus 5DNA. (a), example of typical staining pattern of cells transformed by left-hand DNA fragments greater than 10% of the viral genome. (b), atypical staining patterns of cells transformed by the 8% Ad5 *Hsu*I G fragment.

at least in the early passages after isolation, and stop growing at relative-ly low saturation densities. This is illustrated in Figure 3, in which the growth curves of a number of transformed cell lines of the three categories are compared. Another characteristic property of E frag-ment transformed cells is that they have a somewhat fibroblastic

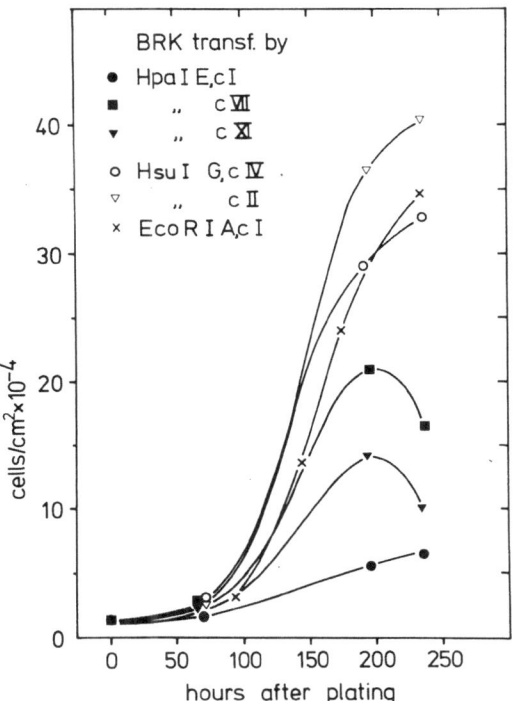

Figure 3. Growth curves of a number of adenovirus 5 DNA fragment-transformed BRK lines growing in monolayer culture. A series of replicate cultures was prepared of each cell line in plastic dishes at an initial concentration of 2×10^4 cells/cm². At various times after plating, one dish from each series was trypsinized and the number of cells counted, using a Coulter counter. The top panel shows growth curves of 2 clones transformed by the *Hsu*I G fragment and of one clone transformed by fragment *Eco*RI A. The lower panel shows growth curves of 3 clones transformed by the *Hpa*I E fragment.

appearance and a large cell volume, whereas cells transformed by larger DNA fragments are considerably smaller and more epithelial in character. This is seen most clearly in subconfluent cultures. All three categories of transformed cells, however, share the property that they are aneuploid.

These results suggested that transformation by Ad5 is a process in which more than one viral function is involved. Cells transformed by DNA fragments comprising only part of the genetic information normally involved in this process may show an altered transformed phenotype because some of the viral transformation functions may be

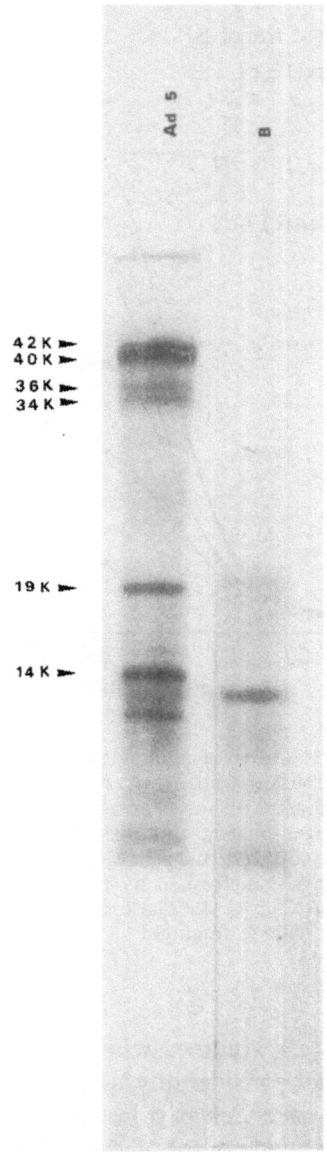

Figure 4. Polypeptides synthesized in a wheat germ cell-free protein synthesizing system, directed by early adenovirus 5-specific RNA (Ad5) or without added RNA (B). The proteins were labelled with 35_S methionine, and were fractionated by electrophoresis in SDS-containing 13.4% polyacrylamide slab gels. The radioactive bands were visualized by autoradiography. (The procedures used for the in vitro synthesis of early viral proteins are described by J.H. Lupker, submitted publication). The proteins encoded by the transforming segment of the Ad5 genome are indicated by arrows.

missing in such cells. Hence, it was felt that a more detailed study of the cells transformed by various DNA fragments could be helpful in elucidating the role in transformation of the different viral proteins. It was decided therefore to study in some detail the proteins encoded by the transforming region of Ad5 and to identify the viral proteins expressed in the fragment-transformed cells.

In order to identify the proteins encoded by the left-hand early region of Ad5 DNA, cytoplasmic RNA was isolated from KB cells, approximately 6 hr after infection with adeno 5. Virus-specific mRNA, corresponding to the left-hand early region, was then selected by nucleic acid hybridization to appropriate restriction endonuclease DNA fragments, and the RNA was translated in a cell-free protein synthesizing system derived from wheat germ. An analysis of the products by SDS polyacrylamide gel electrophoresis revealed the presence of 6 proteins with apparent molecular weights of 42K, 40K, 36K, 34K, 19K and 14K (Figure 4). Since the RNA was selected by hybridization to the left-hand early region, all 6 proteins should map between 1 and 11%. To enable a more precise localization of these polypeptides within this area, in vitro translation experiments were carried out with mRNA selected with smaller DNA fragments. The results indicated that 5 of the 6 proteins map within the leftmost 4.5%, and that of these 5 polypeptides the 14K protein is probably encoded by an mRNA which is distinct from that coding for the 34-42K proteins. The 6th protein of 19K maps in the area between 4.5 and 11%. Since virus-specific RNA isolated from Ad5 *Hsu* I G-transformed cells is translated into the same 6 proteins, it can be concluded that the 19K protein maps in the area between 4.5 and approximately 8%.

Initially, this result was somewhat surprising, since the sum of the molecular weights of the 6 proteins exceeds by far the theoretical maximum coding capacity of the 8% fragment. This discrepancy has been solved recently in our laboratory by experiments demonstrating that the proteins of 42K, 40K, 36K and 34K are related and hence encoded largely by a common DNA sequence.

To obtain more information on the transforming proteins, the virus-specific tumor antigens (T antigens) were isolated directly from transformed cells by immunoprecipitation using sera from adeno 5 tumor bearing hamsters. Cells transformed by the large DNA fragments (> 10%) and cells transformed by intact adenovirus 5 contain two major T antigens of 65K and of 19K (see Figure 5). In addition, a number of other antigens are observed usually at lower concentrations: 52K and 45K, 17K and 15K. The most striking difference with the proteins synthesized in vitro is the presence among the immuno-

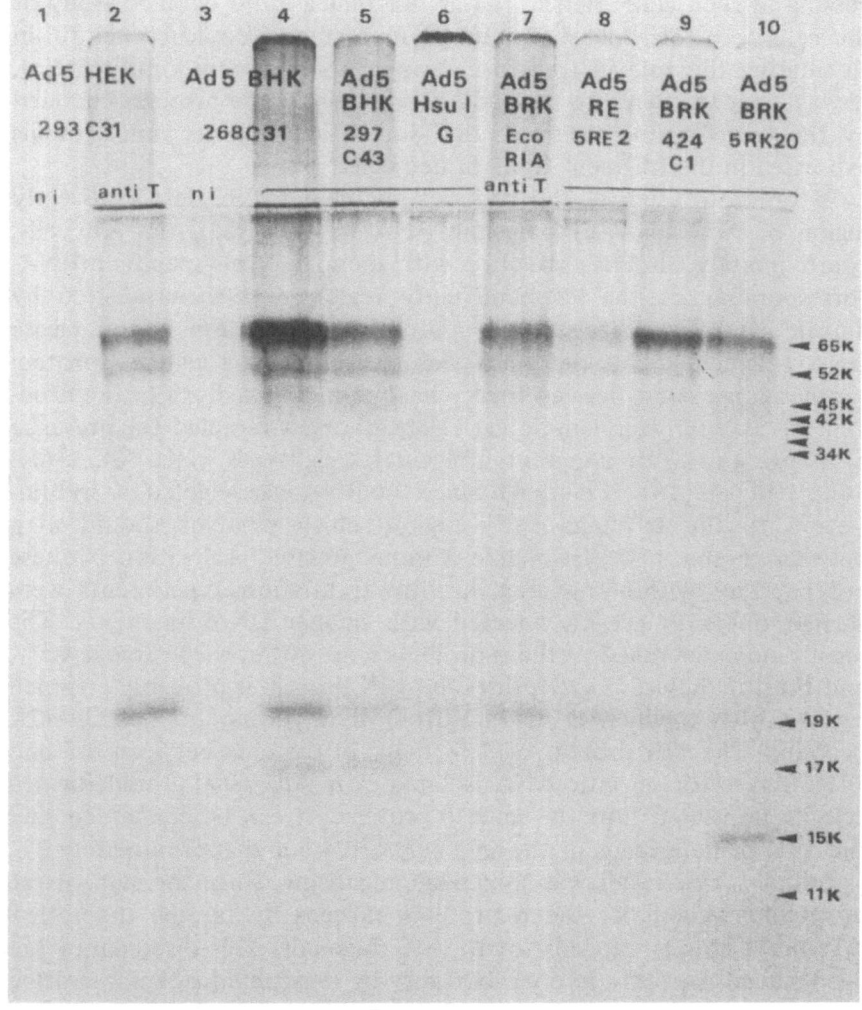

Figure 5. Proteins immunoprecipitated from cells transformed by adenovirus 5 or adenovirus 5DNA fragments, using sera from hamsters bearing adeno 5 tumors. The ^{35}S-labeled antigens were fractionated by eletrophoresis in SDS—containing 13% polyacrylamide slabgels, and the radioactive bands were visualized by autoradiography. The procedures used for immunoprecipitation of viral T antigens will be described elsewhere (Schrier et al., 1979). Lanes 1 and 3: control precipitations, using non-immune (n.i.) hamster serum. Lanes 2, 4, 5, 7 and 9: T antigens from cell lines transformed by adenovirus 5 DNA fragments.
Lanes 8 and 10: T antigens from cell lines transformed by intact adenovirus 5.
Lane 6: T antigens from a cell line transformed by the 8% adenovirus 5 *Hsu*I G fragment.
The 15K T antigen is often missing; the protein may be identical to the 14K protein detected by in vitro protein synthesis.

precipitated products of a major 65K protein (see later). As yet, the origin of the 45K and 52K T antigens is not clear.

The cells transformed by the 8% G fragment differ from the standard transformed cells in that they do not contain the 65K T antigen, but do contain the 19K T antigen as well as an 11K protein. Finally, immunoprecipitation studies of cells transformed by the 4.5% *Hpa*I E fragment have indicated that such cells lack both the 65K and the 19K T antigens (but that they do contain immunoprecipitable proteins of 47K and 52K and possibly a 15K protein). The results are summarized in Table 2.

Table 2. Summary of T antigens identified by immunoprecipitation from cells transformed by fragments of adenovirus 5 DNA.

DNA fragment		
⩾ 11%	8% Hsu I G	4.5% Hpa I E
65K	–	–
45, 52K	34-52K	47, 52K
19K	19K	–
17K	–	–
(15K)	(15K)	(15K)
	11K	

These results allow the following conclusions:

1. The atypical distribution of T antigen in cells transformed by the *Hsu*I G fragment (and by the *Hpa*I E fragment) may be due to the absence of the 65K major T antigen species. Since the *Hsu*I G-transformed cells do not clearly differ phenotypically from cells transformed by larger DNA fragments, it can be concluded that the 65K T antigen has no important role in transformation.
2. The abnormal transformed phenotype of cells transformed by the *Hpa*I E fragment may be caused by the absence of the 19K protein, which maps between 4.5 and 8%.

The origin of the 65K major T antigen species is unknown since it is not observed after in vitro translation of virus-specific early RNA. Recently, however, Raskas (St. Louis) identified a protein of approximately 55 K which maps between 4.5 and 11%. This protein is made in very small quantities in the early phase of infection (this may

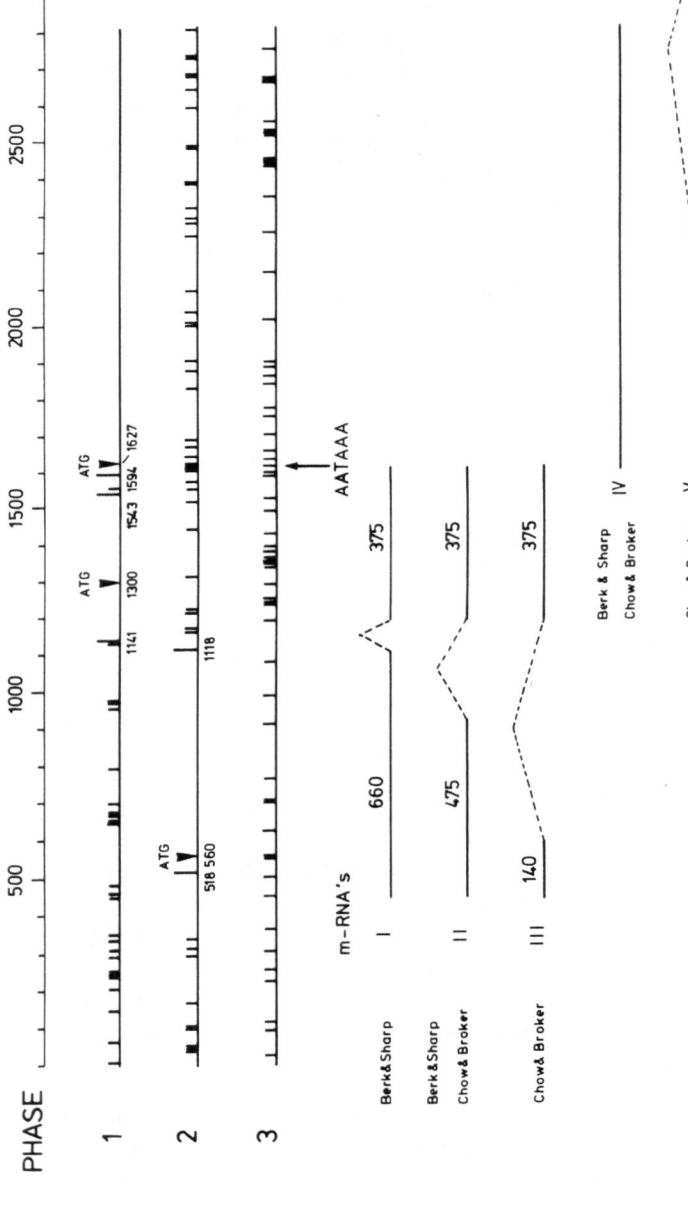

Figure 6. Schematic representation of the termination codons (TAA, TAG, TGA) detected in the nucleotide sequence of the 1-strand of the Ad5 *Hsu*I G fragment (2810 nucleotides; 8% of the genome). They are arranged according to the reading frame (1, 2 or 3) in which they would block protein biosynthesis. In the longer stopcodon-free stretches the ATG triplets are indicated which would initiate polypeptides of maximum length. In the bottom of the figure the mRNA mapping data of Berk and Sharp (1978) and of Chow, Lewis and Broker (personal communication) are summarized; the continuous lines represent the segments found in the mRNAs, the interrupted lines are the intervening sequences which are excised from the RNA in the splicing process after transcription.

explain why we and other investigators failed to detect it), but it is made in larger amounts late after infection. It is quite possible that the 55K protein is identical to our 65K T antigen (the difference in molecular weight could be due to differences in the markers used).

In a third approach, we recently determined the nucleotide sequence of the Ad5 *Hsu*I G fragment which was found to be 2810 base pairs long (Van Ormondt et al., 1978; Maat and Van Ormondt, 1979). By arranging the termination codons (TAA, TAG, TGA) found in the 1-strand of this stretch of DNA (in *Hsu*I G the r-strand serves as a template for mRNA synthesis) according to the reading frames in which they would block protein biosynthesis, we found three tracts devoid of stopcodons (see Figure 6). These extend in reading frame 1 from position 1141 to 1543, and from 1594 to 2810 (and beyond that point), and in reading frame 2 from 518 to 1118.

In Figure 6 we have also summarized the results of A.J. Berk and P.A. Sharp (1978); and of L.T. Chow, J.B. Lewis and T.R. Broker (unpublished) on the mapping of mRNAs orginating from the corresponding DNA region of the closely related adenovirus type 2. Both teams established that these mRNAs consist of segments that are transcribed from nonadjacent areas of the DNA, and that are "spliced" together in a post-transcriptional event. The effect of this RNA splicing can be illustrated in mRNA I, where from the primary transcript a segment has been excised which contains three termination codons. As a result, mRNA I can now be translated from the initiation triplet ATG at position 560 to the stop codon TAA at 1543, yielding a 33K polypeptide, whereas the primary transcript would allow only the synthesis of at most a 20.5K protein, and possibly a 9K protein. Similarly, mRNA II could contain the information for a 26K protein, and mRNA III for a 14K protein. Possibly, the 33K and 26K protein correspond to the 34-42K proteins synthesized in vitro on an Ad5 early mRNA template. The discrepancy in molecular weights between these in vitro proteins and the proteins deduced from the DNA sequence may be explained by the high proline content as predicted by the nucleotide sequence; this would decrease the electrophoretic mobilities of the proteins, and hence increase their apparent molecular weights. The translatable area of mRNA IV extends beyond the nucleotide sequence determined thus far (Ad5 *Hsu*I G), but the established sequence can already code for a polypeptide chain of 44,000 daltons. Possibly, this protein corresponds to the 65K T antigen; if this is the case, it would explain why the cells transformed by *Hsu*I G do not contain the 65K T antigen; more work is

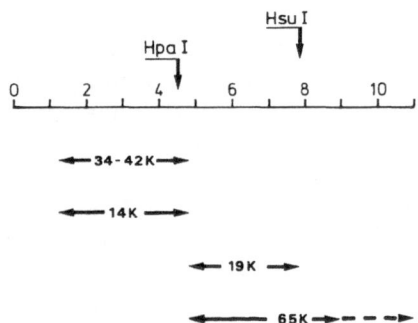

Figure 7. Coding areas of proteins specified by the transforming region of adeno-virus 5 DNA. The localization of the 65K protein is still speculative. The results are based on in vitro translation experiments and on immunoprecipitation studies of T antigens from transformed cells.

needed, however, to test this hypothesis. Finally, mRNA V has space for a 19K protein.

Figure 7 summarizes our results on the localization of the coding areas of the various Ad5 transformation proteins (speculative for the 65K protein). It can be seen that the transforming area is divided into two parts: 0–4.5%, and 4.5–11%, each of which codes for two or more partially overlapping proteins. The part between 0 and 4.5% represents the smallest transforming fragment; it contains information for 4 overlapping proteins (34-42K) and a 5th protein of 14K (which probably overlaps in part with the 4 large proteins). Our results suggest that the function of this segment may be to convert a normal diploid cell with a limited life span into a permanent line still lacking, however, the typical "transformed" properties. The adjacent part, between 4.5 and 11%, should then code for the 19K T antigen and possibly also for the 65K T antigen (these two proteins are probably also overlapping). Studies with cells transformed by the 8% HsuI G fragment indicated that the 19K protein induces some of the typical transformed properties in the cells. As yet, the role of the 65K protein is unclear. It may act in a way similar to the 19K protein but, in addition, it may have specific functions in the   replication of viral macromolecules. This latter possibility is suggested by the fact that this protein seems to be synthesized predominantly in the late phase of the lytic cycle rather than in the early phase.

In summary, on the basis of studies of cells transformed by various DNA fragments, we have been able to divide the transforming region of Ad5 into two parts, each of which codes for a block of partially overlapping proteins, and each of which appears to have a distinct role in transformation.

REFERENCES

Abrahams, P.J. and A.J. van der Eb (1975). In vitro transformation of rat and mouse cells by DNA from Simian virus 40. J. Virol. 16: 206-209.

Bacchetti, S. and F.L. Graham (1977). Transfer of the gene for thymidine kinase to thymidine kinase deficient human cells by purified herpes simplex viral DNA. Proc. Natl. Acad. Sci. USA 74: 1590-1594.

Berk, A.J. and P.A. Sharp (1978). Structure of the Adenovirus 2 early mRNAs. Cell 14: 695-711.

Graham, F.L. and A.J. van der Eb (1973a). A new technique for the assay of infectivity of human Adenovirus 5 DNA. Virol. 52: 456-467.

Graham, F.L. and A.J. van der Eb (1973b). Transformation of rat cells by DNA of human Adenovirus 5. Virol. 54: 536-539.

Graham, F.L., P.J. Abrahams, C. Mulder, H.L. Heijneker, S.O. Warnaar, F.A.J. de Vries, W. Fiers and A.J. van der Eb (1974a). Studies on in vitro transformation by DNA and DNA fragments of human Adenoviruses and Simian virus 40. Cold Spring Harbor Symp. Quant. Biol. 39: 637-650.

Graham, F.L., A.J. van der Eb and H.L. Heijneker (1974b). Size and location of the transforming region in human adenovirus type 5 DNA. Nature 251: 687-691.

Maat, J. and H. van Ormondt (1979). The nucleotide sequence of the transforming HindIII-G fragment of Adenovirus type 5 DNA. The region between map positions 4.5 (HpaI site) and 8.0 (HindIII site). Gene 6: 75-90.

Maitland, N.J. and J.K. McDougall (1977). Cell 11: 233-241.

Mulder, C., J.R. Arrand, H. Delius, W. Keller, U. Pettersson, R.J. Roberts and P.A. Sharp (1974). Cleavage maps of DNA from Adenovirus type 2 and 5 by restriction endonucleases EcoRI and HpaI. Cold Spring Harbor Symp. Quant. Biol. 39: 397-400.

Ormondt, H. van, J. Maat, A. de Waard and A.J. van der Eb (1978). The nucleotide sequence of the transforming HpaI-E fragment of Adenovirus type 5 DNA. Gene 4: 309-328.

Schrier, P.I., P.J. van den Elsen, J.J.L. Hertoghs and A.J. van der Eb (1979). Characterization of tumor antigens in cells transformed by fragments of Adenovirus type 5 DNA. Virology (in press).

Van der Eb, A.J., C. Mulder, F.L. Graham and A. Houweling (1977). Transformation with specific fragments of Adenovirus DNAs. I. Isolation of specific fragments with transforming activity of adenovirus 2 and 5 DNA. Gene 2: 115-132.

Van der Eb, A.J. and A. Houweling (1977). Transformation with specific fragments of Adenovirus DNAs. II Analysis of the viral DNA sequences present in cells transformed with a 7% fragment of Adenovirus 5 DNA. Gene 2: 133-146.

Van der Noordaa, J. (1976). Infectivity, oncogenicity and transforming ability of BK virus and BK virus DNA. J. Gen. Virol. 30, 371-373.

6. PLANT TUMOURS CAUSED BY BACTERIAL PLASMIDS: CROWN GALL

R.A. SCHILPEROORT, P.M. KLAPWIJK, G. OOMS and G.J. WULLEMS

ABSTRACT

Crown galls develop on dicotyledonous plants after infection by *Agrobacterium tumefaciens*. In virulent agrobacteria a large plasmid which is called Ti-plasmid, carries the genetic information for oncogenicity. A fragment of this plasmid is present and is expressed in crown gall cells. The fragment is called T-DNA and it probably harbours the genes responsible for the neoplastic condition of the cells. It is assumed that the autonomous growth of crown gall cells is due to the activity of the hormones auxin and cytokinin in the cell. Ti-plasmid mutants, which induce tumours with different phenotype, have led to the supposition that T-DNA genes are responsible for both hormone activities.

The neoplastic condition can be reversibly suppressed with regard to the capacity of the tumour cells to develop teratomas or shoots. However, no root formation from crown gall callus or tumour shoots has been observed so far. Using a receptor model for auxin action at the gene level it is postulated that suppression of the neoplastic condition is caused by a regulatory mechanism of the cell which eliminates or inactivates a cytoplasmic auxin receptor and which normally might act at the start of cell differentiation and shooting.

The tumour-phenotype is reestablished by wounding. This is explained by assuming that as a wound response the auxin receptor is synthesized or again released.

1. INTRODUCTION

Tumours not only occur in animals and man but also develop on plants. Etiologically the tumours in these widely different organisms have many similarities. The possibility therefore exists that the basic mechanism of neoplastic growth is comparable. We may be supported in this idea if we realize that tumour growth on plants can arise as in

F.J. Cleton and J.W.I.M. Simons (eds.), Genetic Origins of Tumor Cells. 87–108.
Copyright © 1980 by Martinus Nijhoff Publishers bv, The Hague/Boston/London.

the case of animal cells under the influence of a RNA-virus (the Wound Tumour Virus), radiation and certain potent animal carcinogens. Moreover tumours of genetic origin have long been known to occur in plants (see reviews of Braun, 1972 and Beiderbeck, 1977). Moreover, habituation of plant cells, i.e. the ability to grow in the absence of phytohormones after prolonged cultivation in the presence of hormones, could be considered as an analogous case to the establishment of certain animal cell-lines with a malignant character. DNA-tumour viruses are well known in animals but not in plants. However, with regard to the mode of action of these viruses, *Agrobacterium tumefaciens* might be comparable to such agents. Studies on crown gall, which is the name of the plant tumour induced by *A. tumefaciens*, might help to reveal certain aspects of the molecular basis of neoplastic growth. The totipotency of plant cells, i.e. the capacity of somatic cells to regenerate fertile plants, permits investigation of the important phenomenon of reversal of tumourigenesis.

For detailed information on research into the physiology, molecular biology and genetics of crown gall and *A. tumefaciens* the reader is referred to recent review papers (Beiderbeck, 1977; Braun, 1978; Gordon et al., 1976; Hooykaas et al., 1979; Schell and Van Montagu, 1978; Schilperoort et al., 1978).

2. CROWN GALL INDUCTION

The crown gall tumour is characterized by non-self-limiting cell proliferation. It arises when *A. tumefaciens* infects wound sites. Virulent agrobacteria attack a great number of species and families, mostly dicotyledons; monocotyledons do not appear to be susceptible to the tumour-inducing stimulus of the bacteria. *Agrobacterium* is a gram-negative bacterium often present in the soil. In nature, crown galls are frequently induced at or just below soil level in the root crown, where wounds readily occur. Wounding is an essential precondition for tumour formation. *A. tumefaciens* cells penetrate into the intercellular spaces and into damaged cells filled with wound exudate, and at these sites the bacteria multiply and interact with adjacent healthy cells; they do not, however, penetrate into the latter, but act by attaching themselves to the cell walls, from which a tumour-inducing principle is transferred into the cell (Figure 1). Only conditioned cells appear to be susceptible to transformation. These are cells in the wound region which are stimulated to divide as a response to wounding. Tumour induction has to be accomplished, however, before cell divi-

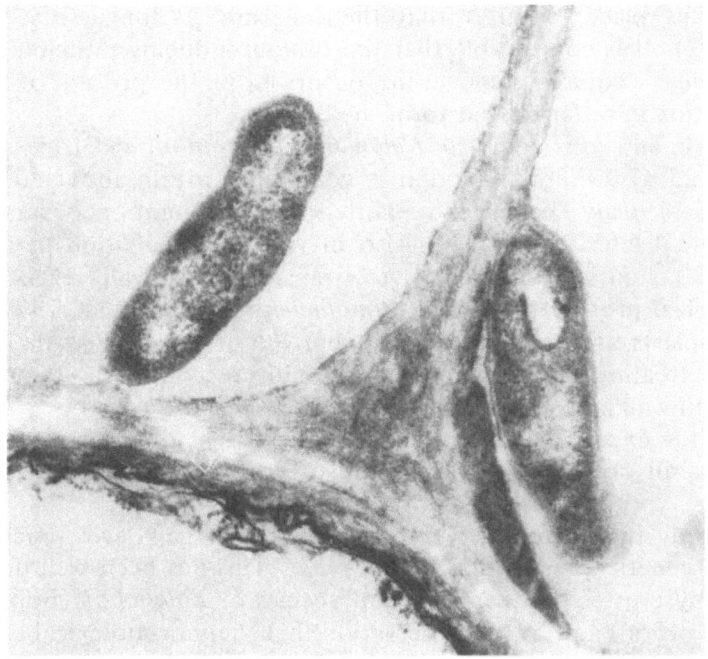

Figure 1.   Attachment of *Agrobacterium* cells to the cell wall.

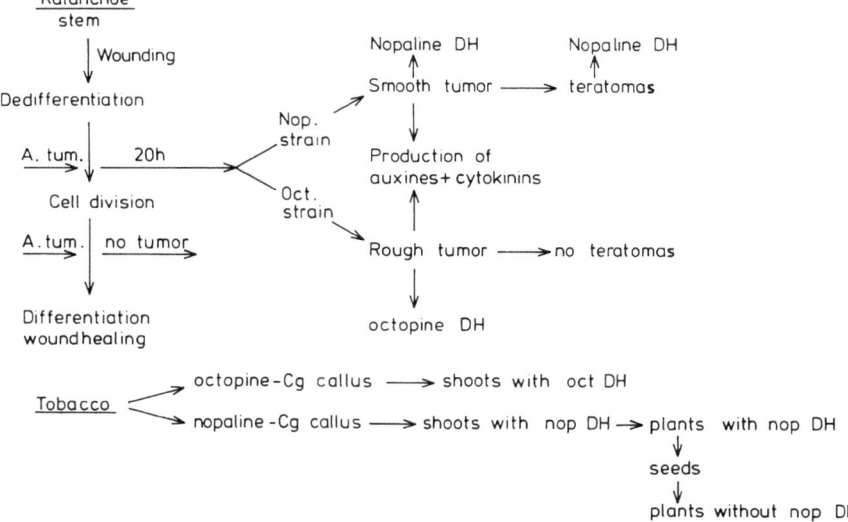

Figure 2.   Crown gall initiation and development.

sion takes place, as after that the cells are no longer susceptible (Figure 2). It is conceivable that the tumour-inducing principle of *A. tumefaciens* requires some event occurring in the process of dedifferentiation in order to transform the cell.

Experiments on stems of *Kalanchoë daigremontiana* have shown that at 25° C tumour induction is completed within about 20 hours (Lipetz, 1966). Thereafter unlimited cell proliferation occurs even when the bacteria are killed. Also in vitro an incubation period of about 30 hours is sufficient to transform cell-wall regenerating tobacco leaf protoplasts with *A. tumefaciens* (Marton et al., 1979).

Protoplasts are single plant cells deprived of their cell walls by enzymatic treatment. Under appropriate culture conditions they form a new cell wall and subsequently divide.

With the exception of the meristematic tissues of the stem and the root tips all organs of the plant are susceptible to crown gall formation.

Not only the bacterium is important in crown gall development but also the genetic constitution of the plant. This has been well demonstrated by crosses between different species of *Kalanchoë* (Bopp and Resende, 1966) and by the observation that the morphological character of the tumour is determined by the regenerative capacity of the host and the type of *A. tumefaciens* used.

3. TUMOUR MORPHOLOGY

Cells of a plant species such as sunflower, possessing low competence for regeneration, develop into typically unorganized tumours regardless of their position in the plant or the *A. tumefaciens* used. When on the other hand cells of plant species like *Kalanchoë* or tobacco, which have highly developed regenerative capacities, are transformed into tumour cells, the morphological features of the tumour are determined by several factors. These are the position of the tumour in the plant and the type of *A. tumefaciens* used to induce the tumour.

Certain *A. tumefaciens* strains induce tumours on tobacco and *Kalanchoë* which develop leaf-like structures or teratomas (Figure 3). This only occurs when the tumours are present on the upper half of stems or on leaves. Such complex or organized tumours are not induced by the other *A. tumefaciens* strains on the same plant species. Specifically on *Kalanchoë* stems the tumour morphology can be used to distinguish between two main types of *A. tumefaciens* strains.

The one type induces tumours with a rough surface and abundant

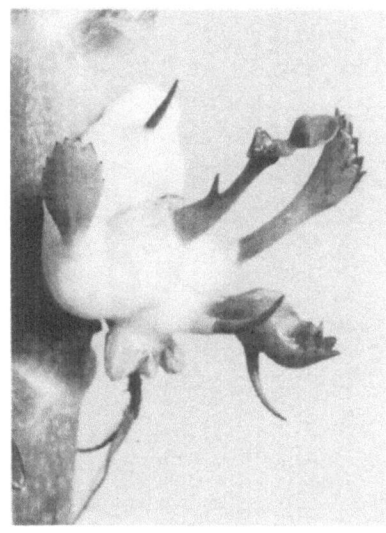

Figure 3. Teratomas developing from a smooth-type tumour on a *Kalanchoë* stem.

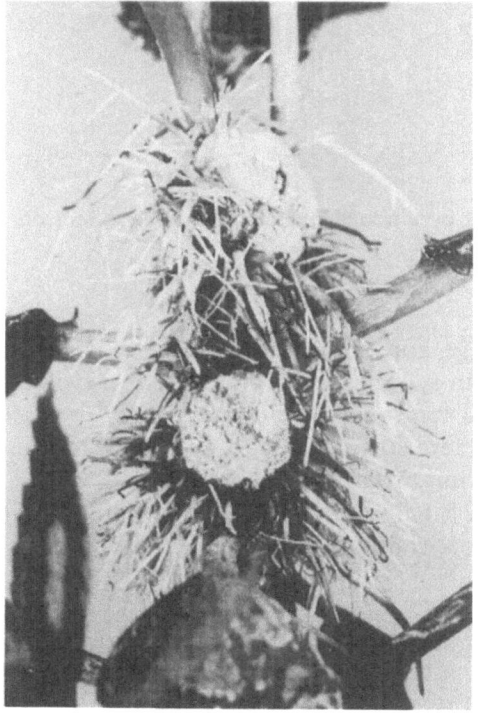

Figure 4. Crown gall tumours induced by an octopine strain of *A. tumefaciens* on a *Kalanchoë* stem. Rough morphology type.

adventitious root formation around the tumour (Figure 4). The second type induces tumours with a smooth surface and a few firm

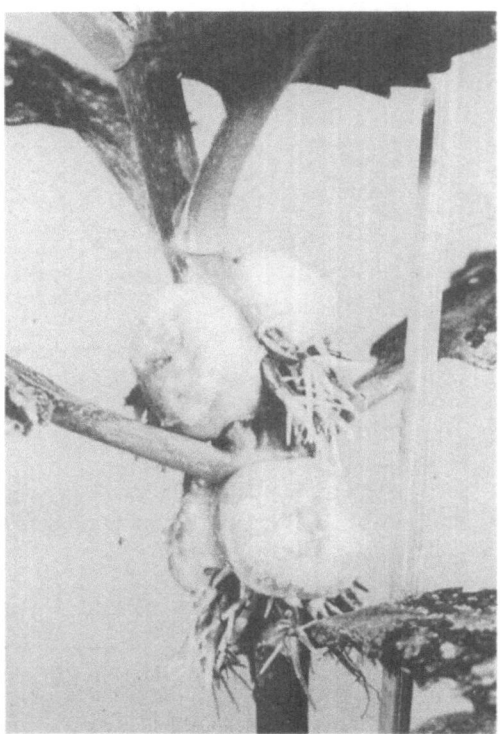

Figure 5. Crown gall tumours induced by a nopaline strain of *A. tumefaciens* on a *Kalanchoë* stem. Smooth morphology type.

adventitious roots, that generally appear at the lower site of the tumour (Figure 5). These smooth-type tumours sometimes develop teratomas. The position effect on teratoma development might be ascribed to differences in the local levels of auxin and cytokinin in the plant. In order to understand the importance of these hormones in the crown gall disease sections 4 and 5 below deal with the physiological aspects and possible mode of action of auxin and cytokinin.

4. PHYSIOLOGICAL EFFECTS OF AUXIN AND CYTOKININ IN TISSUE CULTURE

In plants the growth of one part is closely correlated with the growth or activities of another part. Many plant functions and the course of development and cell differentiation are controlled by phytohormones.

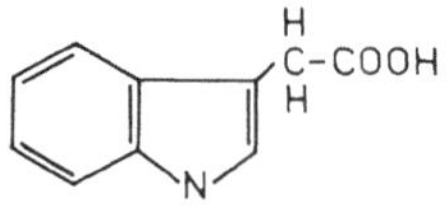

Indoleacetic acid (IAA)

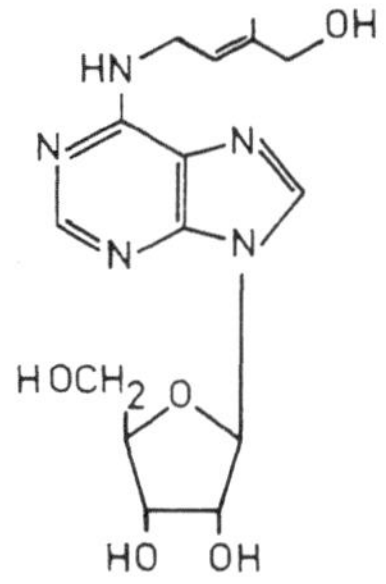

Trans-Ribosylzeatin

Figure 6. The structure of the natural auxin indole acetic acid and the structure of a natural cytokinin, *trans*-ribosylzeatin.

In seed plants five main groups of plant growth hormones are known (see review of Varner and Tuan-Hua Ho, 1976). Phytohormones only partially fit in the animal physiology definition of a hormone.

Like animal hormones the phytohormones are active in small quantities and except ethylene, which is a gaseous hormone, can exert an effect at a point distant from the site of production by means of polar transport. It appears, however, that they can also be synthesized and be active in one and the same cell.

Two of the different kinds of phytohormones, namely auxins and cytokinins, are the major regulators of growth in higher plants. The structures of the natural auxin indoleacetic acid and a natural cytokinin, *trans*-ribosylzeatin, is given in Figure 6.

The induction of cell divisions and the formation of callus cultures from explants of mature tissues of different plant species nearly always require the addition of an auxin to the culture medium. Cytokinin alone is not effective but in many cases promotes vigorous cell proliferation in the presence of an auxin. Cytokinins and auxins act synergistically.

To obtain well-growing callus tissues of tobacco pith tissue both an auxin and a cytokinin are required. For this tissue it has been established that in the same type of callus culture, manipulation of the ratio of auxin to kinetin − an artificial cytokinin − in the culture medium resulted in different patterns of cell development (Skoog and Miller, 1957). If both auxin and kinetin levels were high or low the cultures grew as amorphous, undifferentiated masses of cells. However, a high auxin to kinetin ratio led to the induction of roots in the callus, while higher kinetin to auxin ratios resulted in the initiation of shoots.

In this case and in a few others it appears that these two phytohor-mones are able to determine the pattern of cell development in undif-ferentiated tissues. More generally it can be stated that just as it usual-ly requires the addition of an auxin to a culture medium to achieve callus formation, a reduction or elimination of auxin from the medium is also required to obtain organ and plantlet regeneration.

5. MODE OF ACTION OF AUXIN AND CYTOKININ

The molecular mode of action of the phytohormones is not yet understood (see reviews of Everett, 1978 and Libbenga, 1978). In a number of cases they mainly seem to control the rate of some enzy-matic activities without directly influencing gene activity. Sometimes a hormone, such as in the case of auxin in the long-term response of plant tissue, i.e. dedifferentiation and differentiation, starts such a sequence of developmental changes that we cannot avoid assuming that it acts by altering the pattern of gene expression. Most likely also, plant hormones have to bind to specific protein receptor sites to be active. Studies on the molecular architecture of auxins and cytokinins in relation to their hormonal activity have shown that these hormones must have a well-defined structure to be active. This resembles the stereo specificity by which substrates bind to enzyme molecules.

A cytoplasmic protein receptor for auxin has been isolated from cultured tobacco pith explants (Oostrom et al., 1975). Because it is not localized in the plasma membrane it cannot play a part in the fast auxin responses thought to occur at this site. However, its location is very well suited to mediate indol-acetic-acid (IAA)-influences on tran-scription during dedifferentiation and cell proliferation.

An auxin-receptor complex when transported to the nucleus might induce the need for new gene activity. Such a model would be analogous to the mode of action of animal steroid hormones (O'Malley and Means, 1974). It is conceivable that the synthesis or release of the cytoplasmic auxin receptor is one of the first wound responses specifi-cally in cells at the cut edges of explants. Only cells at these sites will start to divide and form callus tissue.

There is little doubt that treatment of isolated plant tissues with auxin can lead to a stimulation of DNA, RNA and protein synthesis. Evidence also exists, independent of whether the auxin molecule itself is active in the nucleus, that treatment of plant tissue with auxin can stimulate mRNA and rRNA synthesis (Reinert et al., 1977) and the phosphorylation of some nuclear proteins (Murray and Key,

1978). It has, however, yet to be seen whether the hormonal regulation of growth and development is mediated by specific hormone-induced mRNA's and proteins.

Cytokinins have been discovered in the tRNA of many organisms (see review of Varner and Tuan-Hua Ho, 1976). This raised the possibility of their involvement at the level of translation. However, present evidence indicates that free cytokinins do not require to be incorporated into tRNA to exert their effects upon growth. Studies on the formation of polyribosomes in response to cytokinin treatment have led to the proposition that cytokinin "unmasks" a population of cytoplasmic mRNA's which leads to the production of specific proteins. Possibly these proteins are rate-limiting for cell division. Assuming the possibility of a competition for translation between the "unmasked" mRNA's and those already present, cytokinin activity may also lead to a suppression of protein which inhibits passage through the cell cycle. Most of the results obtained so far are in favour of the translational control of growth by cytokinin.

An understanding of hormonal regulation of plant growth would benefit much of the availability of mutants affected in auxin and cytokinin activity.

Grown gall cells appear to represent such mutants.

6. AUXIN AND CYTOKININ IN CROWN GALL FORMATION

As a result of the transformation by A. tumefaciens, crown gall cells have acquired the heritable property to grow on a basic culture medium without added auxin and cytokinin. Crown gall tissue contains higher levels of auxin than normal tissue and also produces several cytokinins (Braun, 1978). It is assumed that this is the reason for the autonomous growth of the cells. The unlimited proliferation of crown gall cells is retained when a small amount of bacteria-free tissue is transplanted onto a healthy plant. The graft develops in a phenotypically identical tumour. This never occurs with normal explants.

The difference in morphology and capacity to develop teratomas between smooth-type and rough-type tumours on Kalanchoë stems might be ascribed to a difference in the activities of endogenous auxin and cytokinins in the tumours. This would also make them react differently to the local hormonal stimulus in the plant. Rough-type tumours show an abundant formation of adventitious roots and do not develop teratomas. These features suggest that they have a relatively high endogenous auxin level (see section 4).

Smooth-type tumours are characterized by a limited number of adventitious roots and the development of teratomas. These teratomas develop from tumour cells, as has been demonstrated with single cell isolates of teratoma-type tobacco tumours (Wood et al., 1978). This character suggests that smooth tumours have a low level of auxin and a relatively high level of cytokinin (see section 4).

In trying to explain the position effect on teratoma formation in relation to the endogenous hormone activities, it is important to consider the polar transport of auxin and cytokinins in the plant. An important source of cytokinin production are the roots (see review Varner and Tuan-Hua Ho, 1976). The hormone is transported upwards into the stem and the leaves through the xylem in the vascular bundles. The apex or growing tip of the stem is a source of auxin which is transported downwards by a cell-to-cell polar transport (Goldsmith and Ray, 1977).

It is conceivable that because of the polar transport of the phytohormones the balance of auxin and cytokinin in the upper part of the stem and in the leaves is suitable for promoting teratoma development from tumours which already have relatively high cytokinin and low auxin activity. This idea is supported by the observation that if an internode in the middle of a tobacco plant is cut and both wounded surfaces are inoculated with an *A. tumefaciens* strain that induces tumours of the teratoma-type a different reaction of each surface occurs (Stonier, 1962). At the basal end of the upper incision a typical unorganized tumour developed, while the other inoculated surface gave rise to a tumour with teratomas. This effect can best be explained by a polar (upwards) transport and accumulation of cytokinin in the wound surface of the lower incision.

7. ANOTHER NEWLY ACQUIRED PROPERTY OF CROWN GALL CELLS

Crown gall cells frequently show the capacity to synthesize one of two types of unusual amino acid derivatives. An example of the one type being octopine, N^2-(D-1-carboxyethyl)-L-arginine and of the other type nopaline, N^2-(1,3-dicarboxypropyl)-L-arginine. The synthesis of one or the other type of amino acid derivative is specified by the tumour-inducing bacteria and not by the host-plant. It is conceivable that during the period spent in the tumour the bacteria actually profit from the tumour specific compounds, since they not only induce the compound in the tumour but are able to utilize it specifically as a sole source of nitrogen. *A. tumefaciens* strains that induce octopine-producing tumours, which always have the rough-type morphology, catabolize octopine but not nopaline and are therefore called octopine strains. Strains that induce nopaline-producing tumours, which always have the smooth-type morphology, catabolize nopaline and not octopine and are called nopaline strains. These amino acid derivatives are not themselves responsible for the neoplastic condition of crown gall cells: a number of wild-type as well as mutant *A. tumefaciens* strains (see section 10) have been isolated which induce tumours without these compounds.

The difference in regenerative capacity, i.e. teratoma development between rough-octopine-type tumours and smooth-nopaline-type tumours, suggests that octopine and nopaline bacteria modify plant cells differently.

The ability of *A. tumefaciens* to modify normal cells into tumour cells is coded by genes on a large extra chromosomal DNA-element or tumour-inducing (Ti)-plasmid in the bacteria.

8. TI PLASMIDS

Each *A. tumefaciens* cell harbours one or more large plasmids. One of these extrachromosomal DNA elements carries genes which are essential for its oncogenic capacity. This particular plasmid is called the tumour-inducing plasmid or Ti plasmid. Ti plasmids range in size between 95 and 160 megadaltons, which means that they can code for about 150 proteins. The role of the Ti plasmid in inducing tumours has been demonstrated by plasmid-curing and plasmid-transfer experiments. When *A. tumefaciens* cells are cultured at a temperature of 35°C instead of 28°C, which is the normal growth temperature, the Ti plasmid is sometimes lost. "Cured" bacteria from which the plasmid has been lost are avirulent and have also lost the capacity to catabolize the unusual amino acid derivatives. When the Ti plasmid is reintroduced into such bacteria by DNA transformation or through conjugation with virulent bacteria they again become virulent and are able to utilize octopine or nopaline. If the Ti plasmid is received from an octopine strain the recipient becomes an octopine strain, regardless of whether it originally was an octopine or a nopaline strain; similarly when the recipient acquires the Ti plasmid of a nopaline strain it becomes a nopaline strain. Apparently octopine and nopaline strains harbour different types of Ti plasmid. Hence one type is called an octopine Ti plasmid and the other a nopaline Ti plasmid.

These plasmids obviously not only carry genes which determine oncogenicity but also genes which determine whether octopine or nopaline will be synthesized in the tumour cell as well as genes for utilizing these compounds. Oncogenicity and the synthesis of one or the other unusual amino acid derivative in crown gall cells are an expression of the presence of a fragment of the Ti plasmid in these cells (Chilton et al., 1977). This fragment, which is not necessarily of the same size in different crown gall callus tissues, is called T-DNA. It is not yet known whether the complete Ti plasmid is transferred and processed in the plant cells or whether only a fragment produced in the bacterium is transferred to the plant cells.

9. T-DNA

The size of the T-DNA in different octopine-producing crown gall callus tissues appears to vary between a few percent to about 10% of the Ti plasmid. In all cases studied so far the T-DNA is derived from the same region of the plasmid. Nopaline-producing crown gall cells also contain T-DNA. Although most of the T-DNA from octopine and nopaline Ti plasmids does not exhibit DNA homology, part of it shows about 100% DNA homology (Depicker et al., 1978 and Chilton et al., 1978). It is thought that genes on this highly conserved region are essential for oncogenicity. A T-DNA and the presumed position of a gene or genes for oncogenicity in an octopine Ti plasmid are shown in Figure 7. The number of copies of the righthand region of the incorporated T-DNA in tumour cells appears to be greater than the number of copies of the lefthand region.

The DNA in between has intermediate values (Merlo et al., 1978). This interesting observation is important in relation to a gene dose effect. In principle, the more copies of a gene there are, the more protein can be expected to be synthesized.

At least part of the T-DNA has been shown to be transcribed in RNA in tumour cells. (Drummond et al., 1977). A portion of these RNA molecules is bound to a segment of polyadenylic acid at their 3' end, which is characteristic of eucaryotic messenger RNA (mRNA) (Schilperoort et al., 1978). This means that T-DNA transcripts are subject to an eucaryotic control system.

Whether the RNA is also translated into protein is not yet known. If it is translated, possible candidates for the protein are the enzymes lysopine dehydrogenase (LpDH) and nopaline dehydrogenase (NpDH), which catalyse the synthesis of octopine and nopaline.

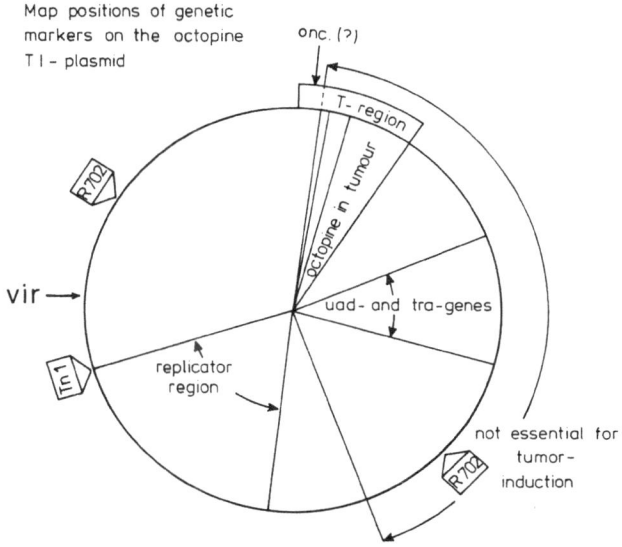

Figure 7. A genetic map of an octopine Ti plasmid. A T-region of an octopine-producing crown gall callus tissue is drawn on the map. The presumed position of a gene or genes for oncogenicity is indicated with an arrow and onc. *uad-* and *tra-*genes are the genes for octopine utilization and conjugation. Vir indicates a region roughly in between the insertions R702 and Tn 1, which harbours genes essential for virulence. Two insertion sites of the P-type plasmid R702 are indicated as is the position of a Tn 1 insertion.

Although it is not yet known whether the T-DNA is present in the nucleus, some data suggest that it is integrated in the host genome (Schell, 1978). The variable size of T-DNA already suggests that only part of it might be essential for oncogenesis. To establish the position, number and character of genes on T-DNA which are responsible for integration, phytohormone autotrophy, influence on regeneration capacity of the cell and synthesis of lysopinedehydrogenase or nopalinedehydrogenase plasmid mutants are required. Transposon insertion mutants and deletion mutants are particularly suitable for this purpose.

10. A GENETIC MAP OF AN OCTOPINE TI PLASMID

Transposons are discrete DNA structures which usually carry genes for antibiotic resistance. They are often present in the drug resistance plasmids or R plasmids which occur in many bacterial species. R plasmids are self-transmissible and because of this can be exchanged between different bacterial species. In many cases they have been found to be responsible for the spread of antibiotic resistance that follows upon the extensive use of antibiotics. R plasmids can also be transferred to agrobacteria (see review of Hooykaas, 1979). When both an R plasmid and a Ti plasmid are present in a bacterium two things can happen. Either the complete R plasmid becomes integrated with the Ti plasmid or, if it carries a transposon, the transposon, promptly passes or "jumps" into the Ti plasmid. A typical property of a transposon is its ability to insert itself in any type of DNA present in the bacterium, independently of the recombination system which normally controls DNA recombination. Because of this property transposons are often called "jumping genes".

The position of the insertions in a plasmid can be determined by the use of certain enzymes known as restriction endonucleases. These enzymes break DNA at specific sites, giving a digest of a plasmid consisting of fragments of different sizes. These fragments can be separated by electrophoresis on agarose gels. Since each enzyme cleaves DNA at sites specific for the enzyme, the fragmentation pattern in the gel is dependent on the enzyme used. The sequence of the fragments in the plasmid for a certain restriction endonuclease can be determined by DNA-DNA hybridization and the use of different enzymes. In this way a physical map of a plasmid can be made on which the specific cleavage sites of the enzymes are fixed positions. Since both R plasmids and transposons have a fixed size their insertion position in the Ti plasmid can easily be mapped by restriction enzyme analysis. This is shown in Figure 7 for R plasmid 702 and for a position of the transposon Tn 1, which carries genes for carbenicillin resistance. By the use of transposon insertions a fine mapping of Ti plasmid functions can be made. Each insertion takes place at a different site and prevents the expression of the gene in which the insertion occurs.

Ti plasmids with inserted transposons are also useful for the isolation of deletion mutants. In deletion mutants part of the DNA is eliminated. Deletions often start at the ends of transposons, which allows plasmid mutants to be isolated which have deletions that start from the different transposon insertion sites.

Studies with these different types of plasmid mutants (Koekman et al., 1979) have shown that the right side of the octopine Ti plasmid, as shown in Figure 7, is not essential in tumour formation. Even when the deletions extend far into the T-DNA, but leave behind all or most of the highly conserved region (see section 9), the bacteria are still

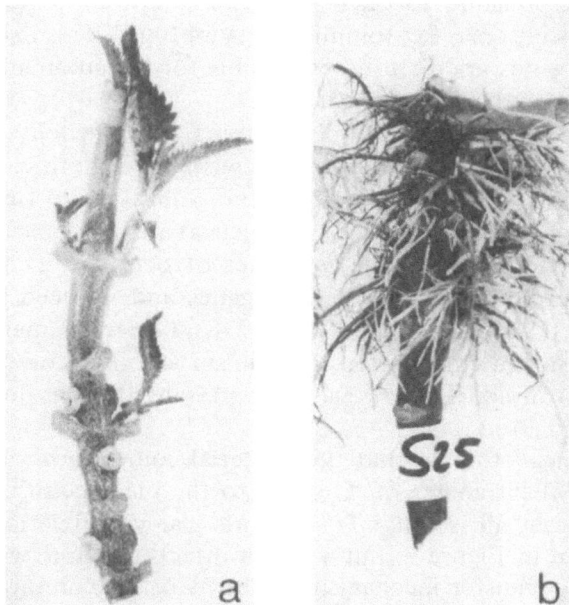

Fig. 8A. Tumours on *Kalanchoë* with relatively increased "cytokinin-like symptoms" induced by an octopine-Ti plasmid insertion mutant. Note the absence of adventitious roots and sprouting of axillary buds. Compare with figure 4.
    B. Tumours on *Kalanchoë* with relatively increased "auxin-like symptoms" induced by an octopine-Ti plasmid insertion mutant. Note the appearance of abundant adventitious roots, while the tumour is small.

able to induce tumours on *Kalanchoë* stems, although the tumours grow slowly and do not synthesize lysopinedehydrogenase. Apparently, besides a gene for lysopinedehydrogenase, genes have been eliminated which promote vigorous cell proliferation. If, however, the highly conserved region is also deleted the mutants are avirulent. This shows that genes on the T-DNA are indeed needed for oncogenesis. The essential gene or genes appear to be located on the conserved region. The presumed position of the gene or genes is indicated in Figure 7 by Onc.

Several mutants with insertions in or near the highly conserved region have been isolated. These mutants gave tumours with a strongly changed phenotype (Klapwijk, 1979; Ooms et al., 1979). The influence of these tumours on the formation of adventitious roots and sprouting of axillary buds of *Kalanchoë* (Figure 8) suggests that two types of genes are present, the one type being a gene or genes

which are responsible for an "auxinlike symptom", the other type
being responsible for a "cytokinin-like symptom". This makes it likely
that T-DNA genes are directly responsible for the auxin and cytokinin
autotrophic growth of crown gall cells.

The position of the gene determining lysopinedehydrogenase is
also indicated on the genetic map. Likewise the regions carrying genes
of the plasmid replicator, genes for the utilization of octopine (*uad*
genes) and genes for conjugation (*tra* genes) are indicated. Ti plasmids
are conjugative plasmids. The *tra* genes of octopine Ti plasmids are
regulated coordinately with the *uad* genes and induced by octopine
(Petit et al., 1978; Klapwijk et al., 1978). Generally many *tra* genes
are involved in the conjugation mechanism and therefore it cannot be
excluded that in addition *tra* genes are present at other positions than
indicated in Figure 7.

It has been postulated that the bacterial conjugation mechanism is
also used in the transfer of Ti genes to the plant cell (Tempé et al.,
1977). However, all isolated Tra-mutants, carrying deletions in the indicated region in Figure 7, but with an intact T-region, were virulent.
Therefore the transfer mechanism to the plant cell cannot be identical
to the conjugation mechanism. The mechanism whereby the bacterium introduces the T-DNA into the plant cell remains doubtful. It
is also unknown how the T-DNA is integrated in the host genome.
Schell and Van Montagu (1978) proposed that the T-DNA behaves
like a transposon; a jumping gene model would be very attractive.
However, one characteristic of a transposon, as e.g. Tn 1 mentioned
earlier, is its discrete size with its ends involved in the transposition
process (Kleckner, 1977). The virulent mutants carrying deletions
in the T-DNA region do not, however, fit in this hypothesis.

Considering the mechanism of T-DNA transfer to plant cells it is of
interest to note that several sites on the left side of the octopine Ti-
plasmid and far from the T-region are also essential for virulence
(Figure 7), for we have found that insertions at these sites cause
avirulence (Ooms et al., 1978). It is not yet known whether the
corresponding genes have a transient function in the plant cell in those
cases where the complete Ti plasmid appears to be transferred or
whether they are needed for the bacterium to accomplish tumour
induction.

11. REVERSAL OF TUMOURIGENESIS

Evidence for the suppression of the neoplastic condition has first

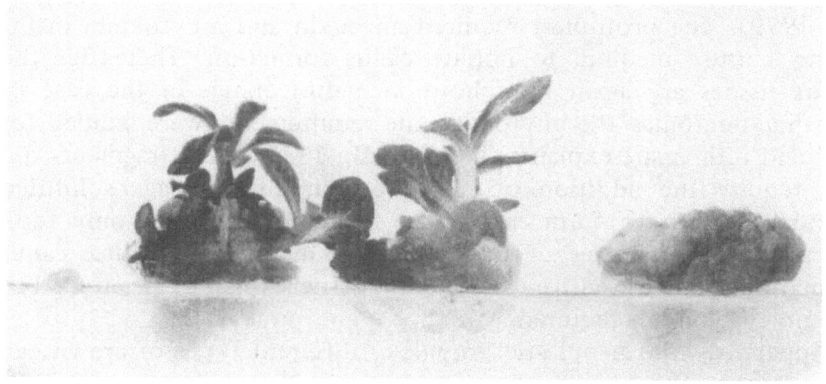

Figure 9. Shoot development from octopine callus tissue derived from cell wall regenerating tobacco leaf protoplasts transformed by *A. tumefaciens*.

been obtained by Braun (see review Braun, 1978). He used teratoma-tumour tissues of single cell origin which were derived from nopaline-producing tobacco crown gall tissues. Under suitable conditions more or less well-developed shoots were obtained. When the best-developed shoots were grafted onto the apices of healthy plants of another tobacco variety some of them formed morphologically and functionally normal apical shoots that flowered and set seed. It was shown that the tumour shoots still synthesized nopalinedehydrogenase, were not susceptible to *A. tumefaciens* (Wood et al., 1978) and contained T-DNA. Haploid tissues derived from anthers and plants of the F1 generation obtained from teratoma-derived seeds after self-pollination lacked both nopalinedehydrogenase and T-DNA (Merlo et al., 1978). The loss of T-DNA may be due to some repair mechanism acting during meiosis.

Although neither octopine-producing tumours on plants nor callus tissues obtained from these tumours are known to develop teratomas, several of the octopine-producing callus tissues obtained from in vitro transformation of cell-wall regenerating tobacco leaf protoplasts by *A. tumefaciens* developed shoots (Marton et al., 1979). It is not yet known whether this has to do with differences in T-DNA in the tumour cells.

Shoot development from octopine-callus tissue is shown in Figure 9. As was observed in the case of nopaline-teratomas the T-DNA determined synthesis of lysopinedehydrogenase is not suppressed in the octopine-teratomas. This was also true for callus tissues derived from protoplasts isolated from the small leaves of the shoots (Wullems et al., 1979). The protoplast required an auxin and a cytokinin in the liquid culture medium to initiate callus formation. Thereafter the callus tissues are again phytohormone autotrophic. In the case of nopaline-teratomas the phytohormone requirements were studied for leaf and pith tissue explants (Wood et al., 1978). Leaf fragments did not require the addition of phytohormones to the agar-solidified culture medium to form callus. The formation of callus only took place at the cut edges of the fragments. In order to induce callus formation from the cut edges of pith tissue explants, an auxin but still no cytokinin is required.

Apparently the neoplastic growth of different types of crown gall cells can be suppressed without suppression of lysopine- or nopaline-dehydrogenase activity, another T-DNA function.

When we assume that the phytohormone autotrophic growth is due to an abnormal endogenous activity of cytokinins and auxin (see section 10), then teratoma development suggests that the tumour cell is able to reduce or to eliminate auxin activity (see section 4).

The reestablishment of the tumorous phenotype in all cases requires wounding and in some cases, depending on the origin of the cells, phytohormones. Callus formation from explants takes place at the edges while the other cells remain quiescent. This suggests that the reversal of the suppression of the neoplastic condition requires a special wound response which only occurs in cells at the wound surface. The endogenous level of auxin or cytokinin in the cells might be less important. Possibly the release or synthesis of a factor by which auxin can act is an essential precondition. This factor might be a cytoplasmic auxin receptor which has been mentioned earlier (section 5). Its elimination or inactivation by a cellular control system which regulates cell differentiation normally would result in the formation of shoots more or less independent of the level of free auxin in the tumour cells. This would mean that if the expression of T-DNA genes is responsible for an increased auxin level it need not necessarily be repressed for differentiation to occur. The T-DNA genes responsible for neoplastic growth in that case might be expressed as continuously as the gene for lysopine- or nopalinedehydrogenase.

Such a situation would be easier to understand than a separate regulation of different parts of a host strange DNA such as T-DNA when it is present as one fragment. The alternative, however, that parts of T-DNA are integrated at different sites in the host genome cannot be excluded. The differences in requirement for phytohormones of teratoma-derived explants or free cells might be due to differences in transcription frequency of T-DNA sequences. Active cell division probably is accompanied by an increased transcription activity, possibly also on T-DNA genes. If so, it could explain why teratoma-derived callus tissue after the first passage in tissue culture is again phytohormone autotrophic.

Root formation has not been observed to occur from tumour-derived teratomas or callus cultures. According to the physiological data from tissue culture experiments (see section 4), root formation is promoted by a high auxin and low cytokinin level. The lack of root formation from tumourous tissue might indicate that the cytokinin activity in these tissues can less well be controlled by the cell than auxin activity.

12. FUSION OF NORMAL CELLS WITH CROWN GALL CELLS

By means of cell fusion different genotypes can be combined in vitro. Somatic cell hybridization with plant cells has been shown to be possible by means of the fusion of protoplasts (Constabel, 1978). Fusion of normal protoplasts with tumour protoplasts from the same species allows the study of the expression of the crown gall characters in the presence of a normal genome. For this approach we used a cloned octopine producing tobacco c.v. White Burley crown gall callus which could not be induced to form shoots under any conditions. Protoplasts isolated from this tissue were fused with protoplasts isolated from leaves of a mutant of the tobacco Petit Havana, which was resistant to streptomycin. The selection of fusion products was based on the properties of the tumour protoplasts, such as white colour of the callus, hormone-independent growth and the synthesis of lysopinedehydrogenase, and on the properties of the other parent, such as hormone-dependent growth, streptomycin resistance and formation of green callus tissues. After fusion a small number of calluses were obtained which were green, phytohormone-independent and streptomycin-resistant. They also synthesized lysopinedehydrogenase and regenerated shoots spontaneously. In this way shoot cultures were obtained giving plantlets which, compared to normal tobacco plants, had acquired three new properties. These are: streptomycin-resistance, acquired by selection of mutant cells in tissue culture, and the capacity to synthesize lysopinedehydrogenase and resistance to *A. tumefaciens*, acquired via Ti plasmid genes (Wullems et al., 1979). These hybrid plantlets, however, still did not form roots. These studies showed that in the hybrids lysopinedehydrogenase synthesis, phyto-

hormone autotrophic growth and the inability to form roots are
dominant characters of the tumour cells. This is in agreement with the
idea that they are due to the expression of T-DNA genes. The regenerative capacity, however, can be restored by the presence of a normal
genome. These results can best be explained by assuming that the
T-DNA is integrated in nuclear DNA, although this still has to be
proven more directly.

ACKNOWLEDGEMENTS

The authors wish to thank their colleagues Paul Hooykaas, Han Huis-
man, Bert Koekman, Frans Krens, Lucy Molendijk, Leon Otten,
Anke den Dulk-Ras, and Lisetta Wurzer-Figurelli of the "MOLBAS"
research group at the Department of Biochemistry at Leiden for their
help.
   The work from our laboratory was supported by the Netherlands
Foundation of Biological Research (BION) and the Netherlands
Foundation for Chemical Research (SON) with financial aid from the
Netherlands Organization for the Advancement of Pure Research
(Z.W.O.)

REFERENCES

Beiderbeck, R. (1977). Pflanzentumoren, Ein Problem der Pflanzlichen Entwick-
   lung, Ulmer, Stuttgart.
Braun, A.C. (1972). Plant Tumor Research. Progress in Experimental Tumor
   Research, Vol. 15, S. Karger, Basel.
Braun, A.C. (1978). Plant tumours. Biochem. Biophys. Acta 516: 167-191.
Bopp, M. and F. Resende (1966). Crown-gall-Tumoren bei verschiedenen Arten
   und Bastarden der Kalanchoidae. Portugaliae Acta Biologica 9: 327-366.
Chilton, M.-D., M.H. Drummond, D.J. Merlo, D. Sciaky, A.L. Montoya, M.P.
   Gordon and E.W. Nester (1977). Stable incorporation of plasmid DNA into
   higher plant cells: The molecular basis of crown gall tumorigenesis. Cell 11:
   263-271.
Chilton, M.-D., M.H. Drummond, D.J. Merlo and D. Sciaky (1978). Highly conserved DNA of Ti plasmids overlaps T-DNA maintained in plant tumours.
   Nature 275: 147-149.
Constabel, F. (1978). Development of protoplast fusion products, heterokaryocytes
   and hybrid cells. In "Frontiers of Plant Tissue Culture 1978," T.A. Thorpe,
   ed., The International Association for Plant Tissue Culture 1978, University
   of Calgary, Alberta, Canada, pp. 141-149.
De Picker, A., M. Van Montagu and J. Schell (1978). Homologous DNA sequences
   in different Ti-plasmids are essential for oncogenicity. Nature 275: 150-153.
Drummond, M.H., M.P. Gordon, E.W. Nester and Chilton, M.-D. (1977). Foreign
   DNA of bacterial plasmid origin is transcribed in crown gall tumours. Nature
   269: 535-536.

Everett, N.P., T.L. Wang and H.E. Street (1978). Hormone regulation of cell growth and development in vitro. In "Frontiers of Plant Tissue Culture 1978," T.A. Thorpe, ed., The International Association for Plant Tissue Culture 1978, University of Calgary, Alberta, Canada, pp. 307-316.

Goldsmith, M.H.M. and P.M. Ray (1973). Intracellular localization of the active process in polar transport of auxin. Planta 111: 297-314.

Gordon, M.P., S.K. Farrand, D. Sciaky, A.L. Montoya, M.-D. Chilton, D.J. Merlo and E.W. Nester (1976). The Crown gall problem. In "A Symposium on the Molecular Biology of Plants," I. Rubenstein ed., University of Minnesota Press, Minneapolis (in press).

Hooykaas, P.J.J., R.A. Schilperoort and A. Rörsch (1979). Agrobacterium Tumour inducing plasmids; potential vectors for the genetic engineering of plants. In "Genetic Engineering," Vol. 1, J. Setlow and A. Hollaender, eds., Plenum Publishing Co., New York, pp. 151-179.

Klapwijk, P.M., J. Van Breukelen, K. Korevaar, G. Ooms and R.A. Schilperoort (1979). Transposition of Tn 904 encoding streptomycin resistance into the octopine Ti plasmid of Agrobacterium tumefaciens. J. Bacteriol. (submitted).

Klapwijk, P.M., T. Scheulderman and R.A. Schilperoort (1978). Coordinated regulation of octopine degradation and conjugative transfer to Ti plasmids in Agrobacterium tumefaciens: Evidence for a common regulatory gene and separate operons. J. Bacteriol. 136: 775-785.

Kleckner, N. (1977). Translocatable elements in procaryotes. Cell 11: 11-23.

Koekman, B.P., G. Ooms, P.M. Klapwijk and R.A. Schilperoort (1979). Genetic map of an octopine Ti plasmid. Plasmid 347-357.

Libbenga, K.R. (1978). Hormone receptors in plants. In "Frontiers of Plant Tissue Culture 1978," T.A. Thorpe, ed., The International Association for Plant Tissue Culture 1978, University of Calgary, Alberta, Canada, pp. 325-333.

Lipetz, J. (1966). Crown gall tumorigenesis II. Relations between wound healing and the tumorigenic response. Cancer Res. 26: 1597-1605.

Marton, L., G.J. Wullems, L. Molendijk and R.A. Schilperoort (1979). In vitro transformation of cultured cells from Nicotiana tabacum by Agrobacterium tumefaciens. Nature 277: 129-131.

Merlo, D.J., R.C. Nutter, M.-D. Chilton, A.L. Montoya, M.P. Gordon, M.H. Drummond, O.J. Garfinkel and E.W. Nester (1978). Presented at the EMBO Workshop: Plant Tumour Research: an Evaluation, Noordwijkerhout, The Netherlands (unpublished).

Murray, M.G. and J.L. Key (1978). 2, 4-Dichlorophenoxyacetic acid enhanced phosphorylation of soybean nuclear proteins. Plant Physiol. 61: 190-198.

O'Malley, B.W. and A.R. Means (1974). Female steroid hormones and target cell nuclei. Science 183: 610-620.

Ooms, G., P.M. Klapwijk, J. Poulis, B.P. Koekman and R.A. Schilperoort (1979). Agrobacterium tumefaciens Ti plasmid insertion mutants with different abilities to induce crown galls. Manuscript in preparation.

Oostrom, H., M.A. Van Loopik-Detmers and K.R. Libbenga (1975). A high affinity receptor for indoleacetic acid in cultured tobacco pith explants. FEBS Letters 59: 194-197.

Petit, A., J. Tempé, A. Kerr, M. Holsters, M. Van Montagu and J. Schell (1978). Substrate induction of conjugative activity of Agrobacterium tumefaciens Ti plasmids. Nature 271: 570-571.

Reinert, J., Y.P.S. Bajaj and B. Zbell (1977). Aspects of organization-organogenesis, embryogenesis, cytodifferentiation. In "Plant Tissue and Cell Culture," H.E. Street, ed., second edition, Blackwell Scientific Publ., Oxford, pp. 389-427.

Schell, J. (1978). Crown gall: transfer of bacterial DNA to plants via the Ti plasmid. In "Nucleic Acids in Plants," T.C. Hall and J.W. Davies, eds., CRC Press, Cleveland, (in press).

Schell, J. and M. Van Montagu (1978). Transfer, maintenance and expression of bacterial Ti plasmid DNA in plant cells transformed with A. tumefaciens. In "Genetic Interactions and Gene Transfer," Brookhaven Symposia in Biology, Vol. 29, C.W. Anderson, ed., Brookhaven National Laboratory, Upton, New York, pp. 36-49.

Schilperoort, R.A., P.M. Klapwijk, P.J.J. Hooykaas, B.P. Koekman, G. Ooms, L.A.B.M. Otten, E.M. Wurzer-Figurelli, G.J. Wullems, and A. Rörsch (1978). A tumefaciens plasmids as vectors for genetic transformation of plant cells. In "Frontiers of Plant Tissue Culture 1978," T.A. Thorpe, ed., The International Association for Plant Tissue Culture 1978, University of Calgary, Alberta, Canada, pp. 85-94.

Skoog, F. and C.O. Miller (1957). Chemical regulation of growth and organ formation in plant tissues cultured in vitro. Symp. Soc. Exp. Biol. 11: 118-131.

Stonier, T. (1962). Normal, abnormal and pathological regeneration in Nicotiana. In "Regeneration," D. Rudnick, ed., Ronald Press, New York, pp. 85-115.

Tempé, J., A. Petit, M. Holsters, M. Van Montagu and J. Schell (1977). Thermosensitive step associated with transfer of Ti plasmid during conjugation: possible relation to transformation in crown gall. Proc. Natl. Acad. Sci. USA 74: 2848-2849.

Varner, J.E. and D. Tuan-Hua Ho (1976). Hormones. In "Plant Biochemistry," J. Bonner and J.E. Varner, eds., third edition, Academic Press, New York, pp. 714-770.

Wood, H.N., A.N. Binns and A.C. Braun (1978). Differential expression of oncogenicity and nopaline synthesis in intact leaves derived from crown gall teratomas of tobacco. Differentiation 11: 175-180.

Wullems, G.J., L. Molendijk and R.A. Schilperoort (1980). Expression of tumour markers in intra specific somatic hybrids of normal and crown gall cells of Nicotiana tabacum. Theoretical and Applied Genetics (in press).

7. HISTOCOMPATIBILITY GENES AND NEOPLASIA

P. DÉMANT and F.J. CLETON

ABSTRACT

Major histocompatibility complex is a set of closely linked genes controlling cell surface antigens, immune response, and complement activity. MHC was found in every vertebrate species which was sufficiently studied and it is involved in a number of biological processes including defence against viral infections. We discuss the structure and function of the major products of the MHC and list a number of other functions of the MHC of the mouse (H-2) and of man (HLA).

It was shown in the mouse that the H-2 genotype influences to a considerable degree the outcome of the interaction between the host and the oncogenic agent (virus) or the tumor. Several examples of the influence of the H-2 complex on the susceptibility to viral oncogenesis and tumor growth are listed, and the genes responsible for this effect and the mode of their action are discussed. Similar mechanisms may also be active in man. There are several examples of association of tumor incidence with certain HLA antigens, and understanding of the role of the MHC in processes involved in oncogenesis and tumor growth may ultimately also have practical implications.

Each vertebrate species carries in its genome a group of rather closely linked genes which form its major histocompatibility complex (MHC). The name of the system is derived from one of its outstanding features – it controls the compatibility of tissues (i.e. histocompatibility). As a rule, animals grafted with tissues of donors of the same species reject the transplants if the donors carry histocompatibility genes other than those of the recipients.

Although the genome of each species contains a great number of histocompatibility genes (H-genes) scattered through most and possibly all chromosomes, the H-genes which are part of the MHC have the most dramatic effects on transplant survival. Therefore, this group was called the *major* histocompatibility complex.

Today we know that the MHC contains, besides H genes, other

F.J. Cleton and J.W.I.M. Simons (eds.), Genetic Origins of Tumor Cells. 109–125.

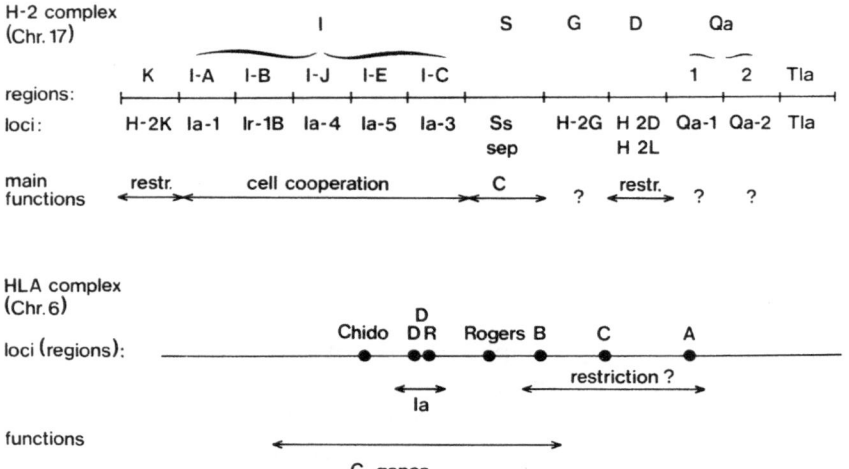

Figure 1. The MHC of mouse (H-2) and man (HLA). Schematic representation of the relevant parts of the 17th chromosome of mouse and the 6th chromosome of man.

classes of genes also. They are linked on a short stretch of chromosome (Figure 1) and control a number of functions. The MHC of the mouse is named *H-2* (*histocompatibility-2*), MHC of man is *HLA* (*human leukocyte antigen*). The MHC of rat, chimpanzee, rhesus monkey, dog, pig and chicken are *H-1, ChLA, RhLA, DLA, SLA* (or *PLA*) and *B*, respectively.

Most experimental data were obtained with the *H-2* complex and this will be used to illustrate the structure and functions of MHC in other species, since the principal features of the MHC are the same in every species. The *H-2* gene complex (Figure 1) contains three main types of genes: *K* and *D* region genes controlling the H-2 antigens, *I* region genes controlling Ia antigens and immune responses and *S* region genes controlling serum proteins.

The three types of genes all have different functions: the genes in the *K* and *D* region are involved in the effector phase of immune reactions against viral and other cell surface antigens (Blanden et al., 1975; Zinkernagel and Doherty, 1975) the *I* region genes control immune responses to a great variety of antigens (McDevitt et al., 1972), and the *S* region genes control the complement activity (Démant et al., 1973).

Other genes, with minor effects or less clear functions, will be mentioned below. The H-2 antigens are transmembrane glycoproteins with

M.W. 45.000 and are associated with a β_2-microglobulin chain (M.W. 12.000). They are present on the surface of all cells. The Ia antigens are two-chain glycoproteins (M.W. 33.000 and 26.000) and are selectively expressed on the surface of some cells (B lymphocytes, lymphocytes, macrophages, epidermal cells, sperm). The complement proteins (Bf, C4, C2) circulate in plasma and body fluids and some may be expressed on the surface of red cells. The biology and genetics of the MHC is described in monographs of Klein (1975), Snell et al. (1976), and Festenstein and Démant (1978).

The association between MHC and tumorigenesis was first demonstrated by Lilly (1964), who has shown that the H-2 genotype influences susceptibility to leukemogenesis by Gross virus. Since then, a number of studies describing the relationship between H-2 and tumorigenesis have been done, and we are slowly beginning to unravel the mechanisms involved. A number of research teams are studying whether similar phenomena exist in man. In this review we shall briefly describe the phenomenology of the MHC-tumor relationship and the features of the MHC possibly underlying these phenomena.

1. GENERAL CHARACTERISTICS OF MHC

The group of MHC genes carried together on the same chromosome is named a haplotype. Each animal (or man) has two haplotypes which may be identical or different. Each haplotype consists of a number of genes, and all the known MHC genes are polymorphic, i.e. they can be found in several alternative or allelic forms. With some genes the number of alleles is very high; this is particularly true for the K and D region genes (> 50 alleles). Some authors believe that this extensive polymorphism is an essential feature of the MHC.

Some alleles of different MHC genes occur together in the same haplotype more often than expected by chance. This linkage disequilibrium may reflect the biological advantage offered by some combinations of alleles in a haplotype. Different haplotypes, and different allelic forms of regions or loci are indicated by superscripts: $H\text{-}2^a$, $H\text{-}2^b$, K^d, D^p, $H\text{-}2K^s$, etc.

1.1. The K and D region of H-2 (A and B-C region of HLA)

1.1.1. Genetics and products The products of these regions are the "classical" transplantation or histocompatibility antigens. The K region contains one locus $H\text{-}2K$ and the D region contains two loci

H-2D and *H-2L* which control the three types of cell surface molecules, H-2K, H-2D and H-2L.

These molecules have the same general physicochemical characteristics (M.W. 45.000 + β_2 microglobulin), extensive similarities
in peptide composition (Hess quoted by Démant et al., 1975) and
they exibit similar allotypic antigenic determinants (Démant et al.,
1978).

The antigenicity in allogeneic combinations is the outstanding
feature of H-2K, H-2D and H-2L molecules. When mice are immunized
with cells carrying alien H-2 molecules they form a number of antibodies against them. Some antibodies detect unique, or *private* antigenic determinants, which are specific for the molecule against which
they were formed. Other antibodies also react with products of other
alleles at the same locus or different loci. These detect the common,
or *public*, antigenic characteristics. The serological entities defined by
anti H-2 sera are called antigenic specificities. An example of a private
specificity is H-2.23 which is carried only by H-2K^k molecules. A
public specificity is expressed on several different molecules: e.g.
H-2.13 on H-2D^d and H-2D^q, H-2.28 on H-2K^d, H-2D^d, H-2L^d and
many others.

The molecules homologous to H-2K, H-2D, and H-2L are present
in all species with an MHC and exhibit considerable chemical similarities indicating that they are indeed genetic and biological homo-
logues.

1.1.2. The function   The *K* and *D* region products are targets for
alloimmune cytotoxic effector T lymphocytes. Although products of
other regions of MHC can also serve as targets, they are often inferior
to the *K* and/or *D* region products in the strength of the reaction they
elicit. The actual biological function of the products *K* and *D* regions
was illuminated by the discovery of the phenomenon of H-2 restriction by Zinkernagel and Doherty (1974).

They found that mice infected with a virus (e.g. vaccinia) produce
cytotoxic T lymphocytes which can kill cells infected with this virus
but not noninfected cells, or cells infected with a different virus. The
specific killing, however, can occur only when the target cells share at
least one H-2 haplotype with the immune T lymphocytes (hence "H-2
restriction"). Blanden et al. (1975) and Zinkernagel and Doherty
(1975) have shown that the parts of the haplotype relevant in this
phenomenon are the *K* and *D* region; the *I* and *S* regions are irrelevant.
Thus, generally, the cytotoxic effector T lymphocyte has to recognize
at least two structures on the surface of the target cell: a viral or viral-

ly-induced antigen and a *K* or *D* region product. Although the exact mechanism is not clear, a number of experiments (for review see Langmann, 1978) indicate that the effector T lymphocyte has two kinds of receptors – one which recognizes the *K* and *D* region products of its own H-2 haplotype (the R receptor or restricting receptor) and another which recognizes the viral antigen (the X receptor). The phenomenon of H-2 restriction is general – it does not involve only viral antigens, but most non-MHC-linked cell surface antigens tested, i.e. antigens coded by H genes on other chromosomes (Bevan, 1975) tumor antigens, etc.

1.1.3. Alien H-2 antigens on tumor and virus-infected cells Some authors reported that biologically altered cells, e.g. infected cells or tumor cells, express H-2 antigens which are normally produced only by haplotypes other than that of the host (Garrido et al., 1976; Invernizzi and Parmiani, 1975; Martin et al., 1977). Although many authors do not accept the evidence and/or interpretation of these phenomena, their discussion may be relevant for some mechanisms of tumor resistance (see below).

1.2. The I *region*

1.2.1. Genetics, products and tissue distribution The I region consists of several subregions (*I-A, I-B, I-J, I-E, I-C*), but the status of the *I-B* subregion and the relationship of *I-E* and *I-C* subregions are not clarified. Therefore this discussion will center on *I-A, I-J*, and *I-E/C* subregions.

Antisera against the products of these subregions detect cell surface molecules, the Ia antigens (Ia = I region associated) which consist of two chains (M.W. 33.000 and 26.000) and are not associated with β_2-microglobulin. The Ia molecules carry a number of antigenic specificities, some of which are private, others public. The peptide composition and amino-acid sequences indicate that the Ia antigens are not homologous to the H-2 antigens (for references see *Ia antigens and Ir genes*, 1977). Although there is convincing evidence that the polymorphism of the Ia antigens involves differences in primary structure (Freed and Nathenson 1978), some antigenic determinants may be of carbohydrate nature (McKenzie et al., 1977).

Tissue distribution is another feature which clearly distinguishes the I region products from the H-2 products. Ia antigens controlled by the *I-A* subregion are predominantly expressed on B lymphocytes and macrophages, and some on T lymphocytes, while the Ia antigens controlled by the *I-J* subregion are expressed on subpopulations of T lymphocytes (suppressor cells). The Ia antigens of the *I-E/C* regions are on B lymphocytes and T lymphocytes and macrophages. While virtually all cells carry H-2 antigens, Ia antigens are not found on fibroblasts, red cells, blood platelets, liver or kidney cells, etc. They were not found on non-lymphoid tumors.

1.2.2. Function The I region contains Ir genes (immune response genes) which determine the capacity of mice to respond immunologically to a variety of antigens. Although the exact mechanisms of their actions are not yet clarified, they apparently reside in the regulation of cell-to-cell interactions of various classes of lymphocytes involved in the immune responses. This was initially observed for cooperation between T and B lymphocytes by Kindred and Shreffler (1972) and the involvement of the Ir gene was established by Katz et al. (1975). The *I* region products are involved also in interaction between macrophages and T lymphocytes (Erb and Feldman, 1975) and T suppressor and T helper lymphocytes (Tada et al., 1976). Some of these interactions are mediated by soluble products which bear Ia specificity. In general, it appears that these interactions involve two cells – one which has a regulatory function and the other which is regulated (i.e. stimulated to differentiate and function, or suppressed). At least two kinds of *I* region products are involved – one carried or secreted by the regulatory cell (the "factor") and another on the surface of the regulated cell (the "acceptor").

Contacts of allogeneic I region incompatible lymphocytes lead to T lymphocyte proliferation (the mixed lymphocyte reaction). Although cytotoxic cells are also produced, in general the *I* region incompatibility (particularly I-A) induces predominantly proliferative response while the *K* or *D* region incompatibility results predominantly in cytotoxic response.

In the HLA gene complex, genes probably homologous to the murine I region genes are located in HLA-D region. Incompatibility at this region leads to strong proliferative response in the mixed lymphocyte culture, and antisera against antigens of this region detect molecules similar to Ia antigens (M.W. 33.000 + 26.000) expressed predominantly on B lymphocytes (Histocompatibility Testing, 1977).

1.3. The S region

The *S* region controls quantitative serum levels of an α_2-β-globulin named Ss-protein (Shreffler and Owen, 1963) and of the sex-limited-protein (Slp) (Passmore and Shreffler, 1970) which is present only in adult males of some inbred mouse strains. The expression of the Slp protein is androgen dependent.

It was shown by Démant et al. (1973) that the complement activity in sera of mice is controlled by the *S* region and that the Ss-protein itself is a component of the complement system. Later it was identified as C4 by Meo et al. (1975), Lachman et al. (1975) and Curman et al. (1975). Presently we know from studies in guinea pig and man that the MHC contains genes for several components of the complement system: C4, C2, BF and probably C3 receptors. Other components may be less closely linked to the MHC, e.g. C3 in mouse (Da Silva et al. 1978). The human C4 component was also shown to be expressed on the surface of red cells as the blood group antigens (Rogers and Chido) which are part of the HLA system (O'Neill et al. 1978). The functional significance of the linkage of complement genes with the MHC is not clear. Since all components which are linked with the MHC can bind and/or activate C3, it is reasonable to hypothesize that the complement genes in the MHC evolved from an ancestral C3 activating protein by duplication, giving rise to the different pathways of complement activation.

1.4. *Other genes within or closely linked to MHC*

1.4.1. Alloantigens Tla, H-31, H-32, Qa-1, Qa-2, 3, H-2T are loci located at the distal (D) end of H-2 and coding for alloantigens expression on thymus cells and leukemia cells (TL antigens controlled by the *Tla* locus), histocompatibility antigens (H-32, H-32, H-2T), and T lymphocyte antigens (Qa-1, 2, 3). Particularly interesting are the TL antigens. In some strains leukemia cells can express TL antigens which never appear on normal blood cells in this strain but are present on normal thymocytes or some other cells. This selective derepression phenomenon indicates that some structural MHC-linked genes are never expressed under normal conditions. Products of such genes could appear as tumor specific antigens on malignant cells (see below).

1.4.2. Enzymes In several species a group of enzymes was found to be coded by genes more or less closely linked with MHC: Acp-1 (Acid phosphatase-1), Ap1 (acid phosphatase-liver), Ce-2 (kidney catalase), Glo-1 (glyoxalase-1), Map-2 (alpha-mannosidase processing-2), Pgk-2 (phosphoglycerate-kinase-2) (for references see recent issues of Mouse News Letters and Histocompatibility Testing).

1.4.3. Other loci A variety of loci with diverse effects has been shown to be linked with MHC in mouse: Hom-1 (hormonal metabolism), Hst-1 (hybrid sterility), T (Brachy), qk (quaking), rds (retinal degeneration slow), Sco (Scopolamine modification of exploratory activity), Plp (plasma protein), Kb (Knobly), Fu (Fused), Ki (Kinky), tf (tufled), thf (thin fur), Low (low transmission ratio), Ir-5 (immune response-5) (for references see Mouse News Letter).

2. THE H-2 COMPLEX AND MALIGNANCY

The role of H-2 linked genes in susceptibility to viral leukemogenesis was first recognized by Lilly (1964) who noted that the inbred strains with high susceptibility to Gross virus induced leukemia have H-2k haplotype. Subsequently, in crosses between Gross virus susceptible and resistant strains he has shown that the mice which inherited the H-2 haplotype from the resistant strain are more resistant to the induction of leukemia than those which lack this haplotype. In the past decade, a number of studies with different leukemogenic viruses using congenic mouse strains were reported. The results show that there are several types of effects through which the genes of the *H-2* gene complex may affect the outcome of the interaction between the virus and tumor on one hand and the host on the other hand. We shall list some examples of such effects.

2.1. *The role of the* K *and* D *regions*

Mühlbock and Dux (1974) reported that the resistance or susceptibility of congenic mouse strains to the tumorigenic effects of neonatal exposure to MTV (mammary tumor virus) is controlled by the *D* region of the H-2 complex. This finding came as a surprise at the time when the attention of most investigators was directed to the biological role of *I* region in interactions between the host and an invading agent (bacterium, virus, tumor). Subsequent studies in a number of laboratories, however, fully confirmed this finding on the biological significance of the *D* region of H-2 in the resistance against viral tumorigenesis.

Chesebro et al. (1974) noted that mice with H-2^b haplotype are able to recover from splenomegaly induced by injection of low doses of Friend leukemia virus while mice with H-2^d haplotype failed to recover and subsequently died from leukemia. In experiments using recombinant haplotypes only those which had the *D* region of H-2^b

had the capacity of recovery, while the haplotypes which contained other regions from the H-2^b haplotype but not the D region were ineffective in this respect. These results indicate that the D region of H-2^b contains gene(s) which determine resistance to the Friend virus induced leukemia. The experiments of Bubbers and Lilly (1977) indicated that the known product of the D^b region, the H-2D^b antigen itself, may be involved in this effect, since it is physically associated with the viral antigens on the cell membrane and it becomes incorporated into the viral particles produced by the infected animal. In contrast the corresponding product of the D region of a susceptible haplotype, H-2^d, is not associated with the viral antigens on the cell and is not incorporated into the virus. Gomard et al. (1978) have shown that anti-MSV (Moloney Sarcome Virus) immune lymphocytes and anti-FLV immune lymphocytes were able to lyse lymphoma cells induced by a variety of viruses (Moloney, Rauscher, Friend, Graffi, Tennant) only if both the immune lymphocyte and the target cell shared either a K region allele of the H-2^d haplotype or the D region allele of the H-2^b haplotype. In these instances the lysis could be specifically blocked by anti-H-2K^d or anti-H-2D^b antisera, again indicating that the products of the K and D region, the H-2K and H-2D antigens, are directly involved in the interaction between the infected cell and the immune lymphocyte.

Meruello and co-workers (1977) have tested susceptibility of a number of congenic mouse strains to leukemogenesis by a virus obtained from a radiation-induced leukemia, and found that only mice with the D region of the H-2^d haplotype were resistant to the leukemogenic effects of intrathymic injection of the virus, while mice with the D region of H-2^s or H-2^q haplotype were susceptible. When they analysed the expression of H-2K and H-2D antigens on thymus cells before and after injection of the virus, Meruello et al. (1978) observed that while expression of H-2K antigens increased after infection both in susceptible and in resistant strains, the expression of H-2D antigens increased only in the strains which had the resistance-conferring D^d region. Thus, a number of studies in different systems indicate that the "classical" H-2 antigens are involved in the response of the host to infection by oncogenic viruses and the resistance to tumor growth. Whether these effects are always analogous to those involved in the "H-2-restriction" phenomena is not known.

2.2. The role of the I region of the H-2 complex

The H-2 linked gene determining the resistance to Gross virus leukemogenesis (*Rgv-1*) is located in the K end of the H-2 gene complex (i.e. in the *K* region or in the *I* region) (Lilly, 1970). It is conceivable that *Rgv-1* is an immune response gene controlling the capacity of mice to raise immune response to leukemia cell antigens. This notion was supported by the experiments of Sato et al. (1973) who demonstrated that some transplantable radiation induced leukemias of BALB/c origin fail to grow in F$_1$ hybrids between the BALB/c strain and those strains which have the *K* and *I* region of the *H-2^b* haplotype. The resistant hybrids produce antibodies against leukemia cell surface antigen(s) named X.1; this antibody passively transferred to susceptible mice has protective effects against subsequent transplantation of X.1-positive leukemias.

Recently, Lonai, and Haran-Ghera (1977) described a gene, *Rrv-1* (resistance to radiation leukemia virus-1) which is located in the *I* region, between *K* at the left and *I-EC* at the right. This is the first clearly documented instance of a tumor resistance locus mapping into the *I* region, and offers a possibility to analyse the mechanisms of effects of this region in tumor susceptibility.

2.3. The role of the complement system

Virions of various murine leukemia viruses can be lysed by complement after sensitization with antibodies or directly without antibody (Welsh et al., 1975). In the latter case, the viral protein p15E serves as the receptor and activator of the C1^q component (Bartholomew et al., 1978). Susceptibility of AKR mice to transplantable leukemia is partly due to their deficient complement system, and it can be partly abolished by infusion of the missing component C5 (Kassel et al., 1973). Hence, the gene(s) in the *S* region, which influence(s) the complement activity, might conceivably affect the susceptibility or resistance of mice to virally-induced tumor. Convincing evidence for this, however, has not yet been presented.

2.4. H-2 and natural killer cell activity

The natural killer cells are Ig-negative Thy-1 negative lymphoid cells which are able to lyse syngeneic and allogeneic tumor cells without previous sensitization. They represent an immunological defense system which can protect mice against tumor growth in the absence of a functioning system of T lymphocytes. Therefore the tumor incidence in nude mice, which lack functional T lymphocytes, is no higher than in normal mice.

Recently it was shown that the natural killer cells are related to the cells which are responsible for the rejection of parental marrow grafts by resistant F_1 hybrids (Kiesling et al., 1975). The gene(s) responsible for this rejection (*Hh* genes, Haemopoietic histocompatibility) are part of the H-2 complex. The actual level of the activity of natural killer cells in mouse strains is different and influenced by the H-2 genotype of the animal (Petranyi et al., 1975). Similar influence of MHC on the natural killer cell activity was also observed in man (Petranyi et al., 1974; Santoli et al., 1976).

2.5. H-2 "extra specificities": a protective factor against tumor growth?

A number of groups in recent years have reported that tumor cell lines and virally infected cells express on their surface H-2 antigens not normally produced by their haplotypes (Garrido et al., 1976; Invernizzi and Parmiani, 1975). Although some of these extra reactions may be attributed to nonrecognized public specificities (Flaherty and Rinchik, 1978; Schirmacher, 1979) or anti Ia or anti viral antibodies, in some instances, at least, available biochemical evidence suggests that the "extra specificities" represent expression of an H-2 polypeptide normally coded only by alien haplotype (Schmidt et al., 1979). Since these extra specificities are expressed on cell lines readily transplantable in syngeneic recipients, they presumably do not necessarily represent a major component in anti-tumor immunity, although they definitely may cause tumor rejection in pre-immunized animals (Meschini et al., 1977).

The most clear example of a possible role of H-2 extra specificities was provided by Martin et al. (1977) in intrauterinally-induced lung tumors. In strains with low incidence of spontaneous lung tumors (C3Hf) they observed that the tumors detected in newborns, born from mothers injected by the carcinogenic compound ethyl-nitrosourea (ENU), do not grow in syngeneic recipients, but do grow in (AxC3Hf) F_1 hybrids. Strain A has a high incidence of both spontaneous and induced lung tumors and the authors suggested that the tumors induced in the resistant (C3Hf) strain express an antigen normally present in the susceptible strain (A) and hence are rejected by virtue of the immune reaction against this abnormally expressed alloantigen. By suitable pre-immunization experiments, they have demonstrated that this anomalously expressed antigen is controlled by the *K* region of the *H-2*^{k} haplotype. Experiments of Faraldo and Dux (1979), however, suggest that the gene responsible for the H-2 linked resistance to spontaneous lung tumors is located in the *I* region.

2.6. Some other experimental systems with H-2 influence on tumor incidence

Dux and Faraldo (1978) observed that the H-2 congenic strain B10.Y/SnA (*H-2*ᵖᵃ) is characterized by a high incidence of tumors of the lymphoreticular system which occur at a relatively early age. This is associated with a high level of ecotropic MuLV in these mice, as opposed to other congenic lines. In tests on segregating F_2 hybrids the high levels of MuLV are clearly linked with *H-2*ᵖᵃ (Colombatti et al., 1979).

Melief et al. (1978) developed congenic strains, which differ from normal strains by the presence or absence of a milk transmitted ecotropic MuLV: B10-V+, B10.A-V+, B10-V- and B10.A-V-. The presence of virus influences the frequency of leukemias, but both the levels of the virus, the incidence of leukemia, and antiviral immune response are clearly H-2 influenced: the *H-2*ᵇ haplotype confers higher resistance to this MuLV.

Lilly et al. (1975) observed in crosses between high leukemia strain AKR and low leukemia strain BALB/c that the H-2ᵈ haplotype is associated with lower levels of virus expression and lower incidence of leukemia.

3. THE HLA COMPLEX AND MALIGNANCY

3.1. Functional homology between HLA and H-2

The general genetic and biochemical homology of H-2 and HLA also indicates analogous function and biological significance. Thus, a number of MHC functions originally detected in the mouse were subsequently detected in humans or in primates. The role of HLA antigens in restriction of T cell killing was demonstrated convincingly by Goulmy et al. (1977). In these experiments, cytotoxic lymphocytes from a female patient previously sensitized by a bone-marrow graft from a male donor were able to kill allogeneic target cells provided they were from male donors which carried the HLA-A2 antigen. Cells from female donors of any HLA phenotype, and cells from male donors with antigens other than HLA-A2, were never killed.

The HLA-D region is believed to be the homologue of the *I* region of the mouse. The role of the I region in cell-to-cell cooperation during the immune response was discussed above. Data indicating that the D region of the HLA is probably involved in these processes in man are also available (Bergholtz and Thorsby, 1978).

Finally, complement genes coding for components involved in activation of C3 are part of the HLA complex.

3.2. HLA and malignancy

For obvious reasons a direct experimental approach to the role of HLA in malignancy is limited, although a number of restrospective studies investigated whether a particular HLA antigen is associated with a high susceptibility to a malignant disease. One of the recent reviews is given by Simons and Amiel (1977). Clear-cut associations were observed between the presence of an HLA-B antigen Sin-2 (Singapore 2) and an increased risk for nasopharyngeal carcinoma in Chinese (Simmons et al., 1976).

Several studies suggested an association between some HLA antigens and the type and/or malignancy of Hodgkin's disease (e.g. Falk and Osoba, 1971; Rogentine et al., 1973). In acute lymphocytic leukemia several groups reported increased frequency of A2 and some other HLA antigens among patients. Associations between breast cancer and HLA were also reported (Bertrams et al., 1975).

Clinical heterogenicity of the nosological entities may be one of the major problems in analysis of such associations. Another difficulty may be due to the problems of typing of relevant HLA products. Namely, it is possible that unknown genes in HLA complex, other than HLA-A, B or C locus are involved in determination of susceptibility or resistance. In that case, the probability of the finding of an association between HLA and the malignant disease is dependent on the degree of linkage disequilibrium between this gene and the known HLA antigen(s). These problems may be largely circumvented when familial cancer is investigated and the segregation of HLA haplotypes and cancer are compared (Cleton, 1977; Day and Simons, 1976).

Another complication arises from the complex role of HLA in the control of malignancies. Some genes in the HLA complex influence the susceptibility to the inducing agens, others may regulate the resistance to tumor growth, while yet others may act indirectly, e.g. through hormonal mechanisms. Finally, genes not linked with HLA may also play an important role, and differences in environmental factors may further complicate the picture. It can be expected, therefore, that a better genetic and functional understanding of the HLA system, together with a better clinical dissection of malignant diseases according to type, stage, and prognosis, will bring to light much clearer associations between HLA and malignant disease. These will open the way to meaningful prospective studies and, hopefully, to the

understanding of the role of HLA in tumorigenesis and its applications
in prevention and therapy.

REFERENCES

Bartholomew, R.M., A.F. Esser and H.J. Müller-Eberhard (1978). Lysis of oncornaviruses by human serum. Isolation of the viral complement (C1) receptor
and identification as P15E. J. Exp. Med. 147: 844-853.
Bergholtz, B.O. and E. Thorsby (1978). HLA-D restriction of the macrophage
dependent response of immune human T lymphocytes to PPD in vitro inhibition by anti-HLA-DR sera. Scand. J. Immunol. 8: 63-73.
Bertrams, J., O. Thraeschard, V. Feldmann and E. Kuwert (1975). HLA antigens
in carcinoma of the breast, ovarium, cervix and endometrium: possible association of haplotype HL-A10-W18 with carcinoma of the breast. Z. Krebsforsch
83: 219.
Bevan, M.J. (1975). Interaction antigens detected by cytotoxic T cells with the
major histocompatibility complex as modifier. Nature 256: 491-492.
Blanden, R.V., P.C. Doherty, M.B.C. Dunlop, I.D. Gardner, R.M. Zinkernagel
and C.S. David (1975). Genes required for cytotoxicity against virus infected
target cells in K and D regions of the H-2 complex. Nature 254: 269-270.
Bubbers, E.J. and F. Lilly (1977). Selective incorporation of H-2 antigenic determinants into Friend virus particles. Nature 266: 458-459.
Chesebro, B., K. Wehrly and J. Stimpfling (1974). Host genetic control of recovery from Friend Leukaemia virus-induced splenomegaly; mapping of a gene
within the major histocompatibility complex. J. Exp. Med. 140: 1457.
Cleton, F.J. (1977). HLA and breast cancer. In "Proceedings VIth Symposium
tumours of early life in man and animals," Perugia.
Colombatti, A., A. Dux, A. Berns, P. Démant and J. Hilgers (1979). H-2 depen-
dent regulation of high ecotropic MuLV expression. J. Natl. Cancer Inst.
(in press).
Curman, B., L. Ostberg, L. Sanberg, I. Malmheden-Eriksson, G. Stalenheim,
L. Rask and P.A. Peterson (1975). H-2 linked Ss protein is C4 component of
complement. Nature 258: 243.
DaSilva, F.P., G.F. Hoecker, N.K. Day, K. Vienne and P. Rubenstein (1978).
Murine complement component 3: Genetic variation and linkage to H-2. Proc.
Natl. Acad. Sci. USA 75: 963-965.
Day, N.E. and N.J. Simons (1976). Disease susceptibility genes – their identifica-
tion by multiple case family studies. Tissue antigens 8: 109-119.
Démant, P., J. Capkova, E. Hinzova and B. Voracova (1973). The role of the
histocompatibility 2-linked Ss-S1p region in the control of mouse comple-
ment. Proc. Natl. Acad. Sci. (Wash.) 70: 863.
Démant, P., G.D. Snell, M. Hess, F. Lemonnier, C. Neauport-Sautes and F. Kourilsky
(1975). Separate and polymorphic loci controlling two types of polypeptide
chains bearing the H-2 private and public specificities. J. Immunogenet. 2: 263.
Démant, P., D. Iványi, C. Neauport-Sautes and M. Snoek (1978). H-2.28 an
alloantigenic marker expressed on all three known types of H-2 molecules.
Proc. Natl. Acad. Sci. USA 75: 4441.
Démant, P. and C. Neauport-Sautes (1978). H-2L locus and the system of H-2
specificities. Immunogenetics 7: 295-311.
Dux, A. and M.J. Faraldo (1978). Splenomegaly, anemia and reticular neoplasms
in the congenic resistant mouse strain B10.Y. In "Advances in comparative

leukemia research, 1977," Bentvelzen et al., eds., Elsevier North-Holland, Amsterdam, pp. 78-83.

Erb, P. and M. Feldman (1975). The role of macrophages in the generation of T-helper cells. II. The genetic control of the macrophage-T-Cell interaction for helper cell induction with soluble antigens. J. Exp. Med. 142: 460.

Falk, J.A. and D. Osoba (1971). HLA antigens and survival in Hodgkin's disease. Lancet ii: 197.

Faraldo, M.J. and A. Dux (1979). H-2 dependent differences in frequency of spontaneous lung tumors in congenic mice. Manuscript in preparation.

Festenstein, H. and P. Démant (1978). HLA and H-2: Basic immunogenetics, Biology and Clinical Relevance. Edward Arnold, London.

Flaherty, L. and E. Rinchik (1978). No evidence for foreign H-2 specificities on the EL 4 mouse lymphoma. Nature 273: 52-54.

Freed, J.H. and S.G. Nathenson (1978). Antigenic structure of the Ia glycoprotein moleculus. In "Ir genes and Ia antigens," H.O. McDevitt, ed., Academic Press, N.Y. pp. 263-273.

Garrido, F., V. Schirrmacher and H. Festenstein (1976). H-2 like specificities of foreign haplotypes appearing on a mouse sarcoma after vaccinia virus infection. Nature 259: 228.

Gomard, E., V.V. Duprez, T. Reme, M.J. Colombani and J.P. Levy (1978). Exclusive involvement of $H2D^b$ or $H-2K^d$ product in the interaction between T-killer lymphocytes and syngeneic $H-2^b$ or $H-2^d$ viral lymphomas. J. Exp. Med. 146: 909-922.

Goulmy, E., A. Termijtelen, B.A. Bradley and J.J. Rood (1977). Y antigen killing by women is restricted by HLA. Nature 266: 544.

Histocompatibility testing 1977 (1978). W.J. Bodmer, ed., Munksgaard, Copenhagen.

Invernizzi, G. and G. Parmiani (1975). Tumor associated transplantation antigens of chemically induced sarcomata cross reacting with allogeneic histocompatibility antigens. Nature 254: 713-714.

Ir genes and Ia antigens (1978). H.O. McDevitt, ed., Academic Press, N.Y.

Kassel, R.L., L.J. Old, E.A. Carswell, N.G. Fiore and W.D. Hardy Sr. (1973). Serum mediated leukemia cell destruction in AKR mice. Role of complement in the phenomenon. J. Exp. Med. 138: 925-938.

Katz, D.H. (1972). The allogeneic effect on immune responses: model for regulatory influences of T lymphocytes on the immune system. Transplant Rev. 12: 141.

Kiesling, T., G. Petrányi, G. Klein and H. Wigzell (1975). Genetic variation of in vitro cytolytic activity and in vivo rejection potential of nonimmunized semisyngeneic mice against a mouse lymphomia cell line. Int. J. Cancer 15: 933-940.

Kindred, B. and D.C. Shreffler (1972). H-2 dependence of co-operation between T and B cells in vivo. J. Immunol. 109: 940.

Klein, J. (1975). Biology of the mouse histocompatibility-2 complex. Springer, New York.

Lachmann, P.J., D. Grennan, A. Martin and P. Démant (1975). Identification of Ss protein as murine C4. Nature 258: 242.

Langman, R.E. (1978). Cell-mediated immunity and the major histo-compatibility complex. Rev. Physiol. Biochem. Pharmacol. 81: 1-37.

Lilly, F., E.A. Boyse, L.J. Old (1964). Genetic basis of susceptibility to viral leukemogenesis. Lancet 2: 1207-1209.

Lilly, F. (1970). The role of genetics in Gross virus leukemogenesis. Bibl. Haematol 36: 213.

Lilly, F., M. Duran-Reynolds and W.P. Rowe (1975). Correlation of early murine leukemia virus titer and H-2 type with spontaneous leukemia in mice of the BALB/c x AKR cross: A genetic analysis. J. Exp. Med. 141: 882-888.

Lonai, P. and N. Haran-Ghera (1977). Resistance genes to murine leukemia in the I immune response gene region of the H-2 complex. J. Exp. Med. 146: 1164.

Martin, W.J., T.G. Gipson S.E. Martin and J.M. Rice (1977). Derepressed alloantigen on transplacentally induced lung tumor coded for by H-2 linked gene. Science 194: 532-533.

McDevitt, H.O., B.D. Deak, D.C. Shrefler, J. Klein, J.H. Stimpfling and G.D. Snell (1972). Genetic control of immune response: mapping of the Ir-1 locus. J. Exp. Med. 135: 1259.

McKenzie, I.F.C., A. Clarke and C.R.P. Parish (1977). Ia antigenic specificities are oligosaccharide in nature: hapten inhibition studies. J. Exp. Med. 145: 1039.

Melief, C.J., A. Vlug, W. Barendsen, C. de Bruyne and J.L. Molenaar (1978). Ecotropic type C RNA virus expression and its consequences in congenic resistant C57BL mice. In "Advances in comparative leukemia research, 1977," Bentvelzen et al., eds., Elsevier North Holland, Amsterdam, pp. 78-83.

Meo, T., T. Krasteff and D.C. Shreffler (1975). Immunochemical characterization of murine H-2 controlled Ss (serum substance) protein through identification of its human homologue as the fourth component of complement. Proc. Natl. Acad. Sci. (U.S.A.) 72: 4536.

Meruello, D., M. Lieberman, N. Ginzton, B. Deak and H.O. McDevitt (1977). Genetic control or radiation-leukemia virus induced tumorigenesis-I. Role of the major histocompatibility complex H-2. J. Exp. Med. 146: 1088.

Meruello, D., S.H. Nimelstein, P.P. Jones, M. Lieberman and H.O. McDevitt (1978). Increased synthesis and expression of H-2 antigens on thumocytes as a result of radiation leukemia virus injection: a possible mechanism for H-2 linked control of virus-induced neoplasia. J. Exp. Med. 147: 470-487.

Meschini, A., G. Invernizzi and G. Parmiani (1977). Expression of alien H-2 specificities on a chemically induced BALB/c lymphosarcoma. Int. J. Cancer 20: 271-283.

Mühlbock, O. and A. Dux (1974). Histocompatibility genes (the H-2 complex) and susceptibility to mammary tumour virus in mice. J. Nat. Cancer Inst. 53: 993.

O'Neill, G.J., S.Y. Yang, J. Tegoli, R. Berger and B. Dupont (1978). Chido and Roger blood groups are distinct antigenic components of human complement C4. Nature 273: 668-670.

Passmore, H.C. and D.C. Shreffler (1970). A sex limited serum protein variant in the mouse: inheritance and association with the H-2 region. Biochem. Genet. 4: 351.

Petrányi, G., M. Benczur, C.E. Onody and S.R. Hollan (1974). HLA-3, 7 and lymphocyte cytotoxic activity. Lancet 1: 736.

Rogentine, G.N., R.J. Trappani and R.A. Yankee (1973). HLA antigens and acute lymphocytic leukemia. The nature of the HLA-A2 association. Tissue antigens 3: 470.

Sato, H., E.A. Boyse, T. Aoki, C. Iritani and L.J. Old (1973). Leukemia associated transplantation antigens related to murine leukemia virus. The X.1 system: Immune response controlled by a locus linked to H-2. J. Exp. Med. 138: 593-606.

Santoli, D., G. Trinchieri, C.M. Zmijewski and H. Koprowski (1976). HLA-related control of spontaneous and antibody-dependent cell-mediated cytotoxic activity in humans. J. Immunol. 117: 765-770.

Schirmacher, V. (1979). Characterization of antigens of murine tumor cells reacting with alloantisera against foreign H-2 specificities. Z. Immunitäts F. (in press).

Schmidt W. and H. Festenstein (1980). Serological and immunochemical studies of H-2 allospecificities on K36, a syngeneic tumour of AKR. J. Immunogenetcs (in press).

Shreffler, D.C. and R.D. Owen (1963). A serologically detected variant in mouse serum. Inheritance and association with the histocompatibility 2-locus. Genetics 48: 9.

Simons, M.J., G.B. Wee, E.H. Goh, S.H. Chan, K. Shanmugaratnam, N.E. Day and G. de Thé (1976). Immunogenetic aspects of nasopharyngeal carcinoma. IV. Increased risk in Chinese for nasopharyngeal carcinoma associated with a Chinese related HLA-profile (A2, Singapore-2). J. Natl. Cancer Inst. 57: 977.

Simons, M.J. and J.L. Amiel (1977). HLA and Malignant diseases. In "HLA and Disease," J. Daussel and A. Svejgaard, eds., Munksgaard, Copenhagen, pp. 212-232.

Snell, G.D., J. Dausset and S.G. Nathenson (1978). Histocompatibility. Academic Press, New York.

Tada, T., M. Taniguchi and C.S. David (1976). Properties of the antigen specific suppressive T cell factor in the regulation of antibody response of the mouse. IV. Special subregion assignment of the gene (S) that codes for the suppressive T cell factor in the H-2 histocompatibility complex. J. Exp. Med. 144: 713.

Welsh, R.M., N.R. Cooper, F.C. Jensen and M.B.A. Oldstone (1975). Human serum lyses RNA tumor viruses. Nature 257: 612.

Zinkernagel, R.M. and P.C. Doherty (1974). Restriction of in vitro T cellmediated cytotoxicity in lymphocytic choriomeningitis within a syngeneic or allogeneic system. Nature 248: 701.

Zinkernagel, R.M. and P.C. Doherty (1975). H-2 compatibility requirement for T cell-mediated lysis of target cells infected with lymphocyte choriomeningitis virus. Different cytotoxic specificities associated with structures coded for in H-2K or H-2D. J. Exp. Med. 141: 1427-1436.

SUBJECT INDEX

adenovirus 5DNA
  nucleotide sequence 82, 83
  restriction endonuclease fragments
    74, 79
  transforming activity 74
adenovirus 5 mRNA
  encoded proteins 78, 79
  purification 79
  in vitro translation 78, 79
adenovirus 5 T antigens
  coding areas 84
  immunoprecipitation 80 81
adventitious roots 95
Agrobacterium tumefaciens 87, 88
alkylation 28
antibodies 61
antigens
  adenovirus 5 T 84
  H-2 117
  public antigenic determinants 113
  private antigenic determinants
    112, 113
  tumour specific 115
Ataxia telangiectasia 29, 33
autonomous growth 87
auxin 92, 93
auxin-like symptom 102

β-microglobulin 111
bypass repair 37

C-type oncovirus 64, 65
calcium technique 74
Cancers
  acute lymphocytic leukemia 121
  carcinoma 54
  frog carcinoma 16
  Hodgkin's disease 121
  human breast cancer 53, 54
  leukemia 54, 60, 61, 64
  lymphoma 54
  sarcoma 55

teratocarcinoma 17
teratoma 90, 96
carcinogenicity 11
carcinogenic potency 20
chromosome aberrations 15
chromosomal structure 31, 33
complement 110, 111, 115, 118,
  121
contact inhibition 2
crown galls 87, 88
  rough-type tumour 90, 95
  smooth-type tumour 91, 92, 95
cytokinin 92, 93, 94
cytokinin-like symptom 102
cytoplasmic environmental factors 17

dedifferentiation 94
differentiation 94, 104
DNA-damage 26
DNA-polymerase III 37
DNA-repair disorders 29
DNA-replicative fidelity 38
DNA-strand discrimination 39

ecotropic growth 64
endogenous C-type oncovirus 65
endogenous virus 62, 64
environmental chemicals 11
environmental factors 12, 20
epidemiological studies 12, 25
epistatic gene 63
error-avoidance mechanism 38
error-free repair pathways 26, 27
exogenous virus 59, 60, 62

familial cancer 121
Fanconi's anemia 29, 34
fusion 17, 105

gene-dose effect 98
gene products
  precursor protein 59